Epidemic Risk Analysis and Assessment in Transport Services

Epidemic Risk Analysis and Assessment in Transport Services

COVID-19 and Other Viruses

Rafał Burdzik

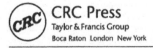

CRC Press
Taylor & Francis Group
Boca Raton London New York

CRC Press is an imprint of the
Taylor & Francis Group, an **informa** business

First edition published 2022
by CRC Press
6000 Broken Sound Parkway NW, Suite 300, Boca Raton, FL 33487-2742

and by CRC Press
2 Park Square, Milton Park, Abingdon, Oxon OX14 4RN

Library of Congress Cataloging-in-Publication Data
Names: Burdzik, Rafał, author.
Title: Epidemic risk analysis and assessment in transport
services : COVID-19 and other viruses / Rafał Burdzik.
Description: First edition. | Boca Raton, FL: CRC Press, 2022. |
Includes bibliographical references and index.
Identifiers: LCCN 2021017618 (print) | LCCN 2021017619 (ebook) |
ISBN 9781032069616 (hardback) | ISBN 9781032069623 (paperback) |
ISBN 9781003204732 (ebook)
Subjects: LCSH: Transportation–Viruses–Risk assessment. |
Transportation–Health aspects. | Health risk assessment. |
COVID-19 (Disease)–Prevention. | Virus diseases–Prevention. |
Communicable diseases–Prevention.
Classification: LCC HE147.5 .B76 2022 (print) |
LCC HE147.5 (ebook) | DDC 362.1969/1–dc23
LC record available at https://lccn.loc.gov/2021017618
LC ebook record available at https://lccn.loc.gov/2021017619

ISBN: 978-1-032-06961-6 (hbk)
ISBN: 978-1-032-06962-3 (pbk)
ISBN: 978-1-003-20473-2 (ebk)

DOI: 10.1201/9781003204732

Typeset in Sabon
by Newgen Publishing UK

Contents

Preface

In order to improve anything, you must first be aware that something is wrong.
In order to feel safe, you must be aware of the risk at hand.

The reality surrounding people changes perception, while perception changes awareness and behaviour. That is precisely what happened when the world was struck by yet another pandemic, this time of truly global reach and consequences – the coronavirus pandemic. Starting from December 2019, the world has begun to change drastically and irreversibly. The initial cases of the severe acute respiratory syndrome coronavirus 2 (SARS-CoV-2) virus infection as well as the lightning speed of worldwide propagation of the epidemic, and so of COVID-19 disease, altered the perception, awareness and behaviour of billions of people, especially with regard to the matters of safety. No one could remain indifferent to this problem, or at least no one should. It was at that time when, completely overwhelmed by the mass of thoughts and emotions, spanning those of fear for my loved ones, responsibility as a father and a son, and determination to fight, an idea of objective observation and scientific research was conceived in my mind. The fear turned into a need for observation, and the responsibility – into determination and diligence in scientific pursuit. I realised that the true value of a scientist is that of social utility, and asked myself when, if not now, the society and the whole civilisation would be in more dire need.

On account of my field of expertise and scientific interest, namely, transport, that is the sphere on which I focused in my investigations. Another argument for such an attitude was the role of transport in terms of mobility perceived as a significant factor in the spread of any epidemics. The coronavirus pandemic has changed the general approach to transport-associated safety, and as of 2020, nearly everyone now understands safe transport as transport devoid of the viral infection risk. However, in order to feel safe, one must first gain awareness of the imminent risk. All of the foregoing has led me to this point, where I can present you with my monograph concerning a comprehensive method for assessment of transport-associated epidemic risk. The challenge I faced involved an immediate necessity of analysing the entire sector of transport services by taking both passenger and freight transport into consideration, which represents a novel approach to infection risk estimation. I hope that the detailed descriptions of the methods designed and the numerous case studies provided in the monograph will make this publication an inspiration and a source of knowledge for other scientists preoccupied with similar problems. Working together, we can do as much as possible to help and become genuinely useful, society- or maybe even civilisation-wise. Everyone can use their knowledge to make one's own contribution, which may turn into a milestone in the path paved towards safe future.

"What makes this publication stand out from other texts focusing on a similar body of problems – is that it represents an inherently difficult attempt to assess the risk of infection in various transport processes.

… Accurate and fully explicit mathematical models and derivations make the proposed method truly universal irrespective of the geographical location and the kind of virus epidemic."

Prof. Minvydas Ragulskis
Department of Mathematical Modelling,
Kaunas University of Technology, Lithuania

"In the current world situation and with the current epidemic threats, it should be clearly stated that the reviewed monograph will have a very large and, what is equally important, almost instant impact and contribution to science in several areas."

Prof. Maosen Cao
Department of Engineering Mechanics,
Hohai University, China

Acknowledgements

I would like to express my deepest gratitude for trusting in my vision and concept as well as for the invested time and energy to my collaborating graduands with whom I was implementing the problem-based learning (PBL) project as well as to my fellow engineers: Wiktoria Lisowiec, Karolina Kurek, Julia Płoszaj, Julia Solarska and Kinga Harasymiuk. I would also like to thank my dear colleague Ireneusz Celiński, PhD Eng., for the creative discussions and excellent cooperation.

My expressions of deepest gratitude for always being there for me on my scientific path and for supporting me in my everyday life go to my beloved wife, Marta, and to my wonderful and lovely children, Andrzej and Alicja, for making every single day brighter and for giving me the ultimate life purpose.

And last but definitely not least, I would like to thank and pay homage to my beloved parents for having magically and inexplicably made me feel like a good human being.

Reviewers

Prof. Minvydas Ragulskis

Department of Mathematical Modelling, Kaunas University of Technology, Lithuania

Prof. Maosen Caco

Department of Engineering Mechanics, Hohai University, China

About the Author

Rafał Burdzik is a professor in the Faculty of Transport and Aviation Engineering at Silesian University of Technology, Poland and visiting lecturer at many European Universities with more than 20 years of transport research experience. He is an author or co-author of books and more than 400 scientific papers, and an editorial board member for several high-level scientific journals and active member of numerous scientific associations, editorial boards and committees. He is a well-recognised international expert in transport, mechanical engineering, transport safety and environmental issues.

Glossary

AHP analytic hierarchy process method

Airborne transmission it refers to the presence of microbes within droplet nuclei, which are generally considered to be particles of < 5 μm in diameter, and which result from the evaporation of larger droplets or exist within dust particles

CFR case fatality rate

Chain of events all activities including the potential virus transmission mechanisms

Contact surface transmission surface transmission of viruses deposited on surfaces from either exhalations or hand contact

Contaminated surfaces transmission transmission through contaminated (by a previous passenger) surfaces

COVID-19 Coronavirus disease 2019

DHI deep hazard identification methodology

Droplet transmission air transmission of viruses in droplets exhaled. It occurs when a person is in close contact (within 1–2 m) with someone who displays respiratory symptoms (e.g. coughing or sneezing)

Effects of infection case fatality rate for a specific group of transport services as the potential total number of persons who have died due to being infected with the SARS-CoV-2 virus while participating in a transport process (at a daily scale nationwide)

Exposure to epidemic threats (infection) number of persons exposed to the virus infection in transport services

Hazard any source of potential harm or adverse health effects, can be anything – whether equipment, operations or processes, work methods or practices

Hazard state vector multivalent vector of the hazard state of a transport service, which is standardised in terms of elementary values and size

HEPA high efficiency particulate air (filter)

I_a daily indicator of active virus infection cases

IFR infection fatality rate

Intervention (restriction)   actions to reduce mass infections (e.g. lock down, wearing mask, social distance)

Kaplan–Meier method   method of survival analysis of cumulative distribution of survival, estimate the probability of survival, and establish the risk of death

Matrix of hazard assessment   collection of state vectors for a selected group of transport services

M_{fa} age-specific mortality factor computed for each of the predefined age groups

M_i mortality indicator, total mortality factor as representative statistical measure of the number of potential fatalities among those participating in a transport process nationwide

M_t total mortality rate, potential total number of persons who have died due to being infected with the SARS-CoV-2 virus while participating in a transport process

Number of exposed persons   number of persons involved in a chain of events within a certain unit of time of process implementation (at a single service scale)

Overall probability of infection   infection probability of the given transport service adjusted for daily indicator of active cases (active infections across the population)

Probability of viral pathogen transmission   probability of the pathogen transmission, without taking into account the individual immunity of the human body

QMRA   quantitative microbial risk assessment

R_{ei} multiplicative coefficient assumed as the measure of the epidemic risk assessment for isolated transport services

Reproduction rate   average number of secondary infections at the given time

R_{eT} multiplicative coefficient assumed as the measure of the epidemic risk assessment for transport service (nationwide)

Risk   effect of uncertainty on objectives

SARS-CoV-2   severe acute respiratory syndrome coronavirus 2

SEIR   epidemic model (susceptible, exposed to infection, infectious, or recovered)

SIR   epidemic model (susceptible, infectious, or recovered)

TCID   median tissue culture infectious dose – method of virus quantification

Total probability of pathogen transmission   pathogen transmission probability of the given transport service calculate as probability of a sum of independent events

Weighting factors   normalised values expressing the mutual significance levels of the evaluation criteria

Chapter 1

Introduction

1.1 PANDEMIC THREATS IN TRANSPORT, THE PRESENT AND THE FUTURE

The global pandemic and the resulting epidemic threats of severe acute respiratory syndrome coronavirus 2 (SARS-CoV-2), which may directly cause the coronavirus disease 2019 (COVID-19), display characteristics of a global crisis that affects absolutely all areas of human activity and human existence. Population movements within and between regions and countries play a key role in seeding the virus outbreaks and accelerating the COVID-19 spread (Simiao Chen et al., 2020; Tian et al., 2020).

Transport, which is perceived as not only the bloodstream of the world economy but also the foundation of human mobility and very often the manifestation of freedom, has also been affected by the global pandemic. One of the most critical challenges facing transport was the imbalance in global supply chains, associated with the economic and trade stability at the local, national and continental levels. Supply chain problems were obviously also caused by production downtime, drastic changes in the product demand structure and political decisions. Another sphere of the crisis in transport is passenger transport, especially collective public transport. This socially relevant transport sector, which has always required balance and compromise between financial result and mobility, and urban mobility in particular, as well as a sustainable transport policy in terms of minimising the negative environmental impact as opposed to individual transport, has faced new challenges. Attempts to sustain the image of an epidemically safe public transport and to comply with the restrictions imposed by state governments often boiled down to reducing the number of travellers in the means of collective public transport, for example, to 50% (or even 30%) of capacity. However, it is difficult to find a methodological, mathematical or sanitary basis for determining such safety measures.

In the author's opinion, there are numerous and very serious problems of the transport sector and transport services which, in this case, result

DOI: 10.1201/9781003204732-1

from the lack of a methodical approach to the problem of epidemic threats, including infection in an epidemic of global reach, all the more so since the current SARS-CoV-2 pandemic is a phenomenon that has never been seen before, and the effects of COVID-19 and the related death rate make it necessary to adopt new measures and scales of epidemic hazard, even if compared to the Spanish flu pandemic of 1918–1920, which was also global and its mortality rate was claimed to be higher, as extremely divergent sources provide, ranging between 21.5 million (Jordan, 1927) and as much as 100 million (Johnson and Mueller, 2002) people. The circumstances of the spread of an epidemic should be taken into account. In 1918–1920, during the First World War, the disease encountered perfect conditions for spreading. There were virtually no hygienic and sanitary rules in place, soldiers at the front line stayed in close proximity in trenches under extreme conditions of exhaustion and lack of strength, additionally deprived of medical aid. Today, the situation is completely different, and so is people's awareness and available means of personal hygiene, a wide range of effective drugs and medical aids for improving immunity, as well as prevention. So why, given such disparate conditions, has the SARS-CoV-2 epidemic been developing so dynamically? The answer seems to be *mobility*, i.e. the ability to move large groups of people in a short time over very long distances. Hence, the enormous pace of the coronavirus spread, which poses such a huge global threat.

Therefore, the author decided to address the issue of the coronavirus pandemic in transport services in a methodical manner. He decided to develop a dedicated proprietary methodology for identification and assessment of epidemic hazards in the implementation of transport services based on the risk management methodology. In addition to the assumed effects of the methodology developed, it seems very important to use it to limit the spread of the coronavirus through transport processes, for purposes of identifying risk factors, selecting security systems and deciding on the method assumed to enable provision of transport services.

People are exposed to viruses in everyday activities, also in different transport processes. Coronavirus transmission is classified under two main categories: airborne virus transmission in droplets exhaled and surface transmission of viruses deposited on touch surfaces from either exhalations or hand contact (Garciá De Abajo et al., 2020). An important and fundamental input to the study of the SARS-CoV-2 transmission problem in transport has been provided in the studies by Smieszek (2009), Smieszek et al. (2009) and Smieszek et al. (2019). These papers describe a formula which models transmission probabilities based on mechanistic considerations, the actual amount of infectious organisms ingested by an individual according to the Poisson probability distribution (Smieszek, 2009), models of epidemics based on the random mixing model without repetition of contacts, the Susceptible, Infectious or Recovered (SIR) model (Smieszek et al., 2009) and aerosol transmission perceived as a major contributor to the spread of influenza (Smieszek et al., 2019).

An interesting approach has been presented by Ng et al. (2020), represented by two risk prediction models for determining COVID-19 positive patients. The effect of each predictor in the model was converted into a score and summation of all predictors that can be mapped to an estimated risk of being COVID-19 positive. A total of 1,330 patients with and without COVID-19 from 4 Hong Kong hospitals were included in the survey.

Given the fact that infected people can travel worldwide and transmit the virus to remote locations, the issue of the epidemic hazard assessment in transport services has become extremely important. Additionally, the conditions of confined spaces typical of means of transport necessitate a short distance between passengers, which may consequently boost virus transmissions. There are five main mechanisms for the transmission and spread of microorganisms: direct contact, fomites, aerosol (airborne), oral (ingestion) and vectorborne. Droplet and airborne mechanisms probably represent the greatest risk for passengers using means of transport.

The study by Mangili and Gendreau (2005) emphasises that, prior to 2002, data from epidemiological studies indicated that the risk of transmitting the disease to other asymptomatic passengers in an aircraft cabin was associated with contagious passengers sitting in two rows for a flight time exceeding 8 hours. These conclusions were based on studies of in-flight spread of tuberculosis, which were considered representative of other airborne infectious diseases. However, a study of the SARS-CoV-1 virus behaviour in 2002 revealed significant differences. In that case, infection was found in passengers sitting up to seven rows away from the host passenger.

With regard to the SARS-CoV-2 epidemic, i.e. the coronavirus, which is characterised by even greater transmission capacity and environmental resistance, the associated threats have become unimaginably greater.

An attempt to address issues related to risk assessment vis-à-vis coronavirus infection in air transport was made by Schultz and Fuchte (2020). The problem of evaluation of aircraft boarding scenarios considering reduced transmission risks was studied. Schultz and Fuchte (2020) implemented a transmission model in a virtual aircraft environment to evaluate individual interactions between passengers during aircraft boarding and deboarding.

If one comes across any scientific papers on the epidemic risk assessment in transport, they are based on virus propagation simulation models or data from epidemic studies. Risk assessment incorporating epidemiological data into mathematical models may reveal the factors of transmission (e.g. ventilation effects). In the study addressed by Ko et al. (2004), the risk of tuberculosis transmission on board a typical airliner was analysed using a simple one box model and a sequential box model.

Opinions on this matter vary to a considerable extent. International Air Transport Association (IATA), in contrast, states that 1,100 infected people flying have been traced and no secondary cases have been identified. The reasons for this phenomenon are said to be connected with air circulation and are explained as follows: the aircraft cabin airflow is downward, the air inside aircraft cabins is exchanged frequently, recirculated air flows through high-efficiency particulate air (HEPA) filters, and the air is quite dry at the cruising altitude. But there are apparently no data that would substantiate such a statement, especially if one should consider other research projects (Olsen et al., 2003; Mangili and Gendreau, 2005). A study on the SARS transmission during the Amoy Gardens outbreak in Hong Kong reported that a total of 40 flights were investigated for carrying SARS-infected passengers. Five of these flights were suspected of probable on-board transmission of SARS in 37 passengers (a 3-hour flight carrying 120 passengers on 15 March 2003). It began a super spreading event, which may account for 22 of the 37 cases of persons who contracted SARS after travelling by air. Laboratory-confirmed SARS coronavirus infection occurred in further 16 persons. The number of secondary cases attributable to that flight remains under investigation, but more than 300 people might have been affected. It should be underscored once again that the current SARS-CoV-2 virus is transmitted much more easily and its environmental resistance is higher.

In this case, the transport sector and transport services have faced very serious problems, which result from the lack of a methodical approach to the problem of epidemic hazards, including infection in a global epidemic, all the more so since the current SARS-CoV-2 pandemic is a completely unprecedented phenomenon, and the effects of COVID-19 as well as the related death rates make it necessary to adopt new measures and scales of epidemic hazard. Therefore, the author decided to address the problem of the coronavirus pandemic in transport services methodically. He decided to develop a dedicated proprietary methodology for identification and assessment of the epidemic hazards attributable to the implementation of transport services based on the risk management methodology.

Chapter 2

Risk Management in Transport

2.1 RISK MANAGEMENT OBJECTIVES: EPIDEMIC THREATS IN TRANSPORT

Risk assessment is the cornerstone of the worldwide approach to prevention of occupational accidents and ill health. The most important piece of European legislation relevant to risk assessment is Framework Directive 89/391, which has been transposed into national legislation.

The purpose of risk assessment is to allow for the measures that are necessary for safety and health protection to be undertaken. These measures include:

- prevention of risks,
- providing information about hazards,
- providing training to workers,
- providing the organisation and means to implement the necessary measures.

While the purpose of risk assessment includes prevention of risks, which should always be its goal, it will not always be achievable in practice. Where elimination of risks is not possible, the risks should be reduced and the residual risk should be controlled.

Hazard, as any source of potential harm or adverse health effects, can be caused by anything – whether a piece of equipment, operations or processes, work methods or practices. The definition of risk provided by the ISO 31000:2009 standard is an effect of uncertainty on the objectives. The ISO 31000 definition of risk shifts emphasis from past preoccupations with the possibility of an event to the possibility of an effect and, in particular, an effect on the objectives (Purdy, 2010). ISO 31010:2009 also describes risk assessment techniques. The latest revision of ISO 31000, Risk management – Guidelines, was published in 2018. Following are the main changes introduced since the previous edition:

DOI: 10.1201/9781003204732-2

- review of the principles of risk management, which are the key criteria for its success,
- focus on leadership by top management,
- greater emphasis on the iterative nature of risk management, drawing on new experiences, knowledge and analysis for the revision of process elements, actions and controls at each stage of the process,
- streamlining of the content with greater focus on sustaining an open systems model that regularly exchanges feedback with its external environment to fit multiple needs and contexts.

These changes led to a revision of the ISO 31000 model which represents principles, the framework and the process, as shown in the Figure 2.1.

The risk management process involves systematic application of policies, procedures and practices to the activities involved in communicating and consulting, establishing the context and assessing, treating, monitoring, reviewing, recording and reporting risk.

Generally speaking, risk estimation methods can be divided into three groups:

- quantitative,
- qualitative,
- mixed.

The quantitative methods are based on predefined measures which determine the probability of the occurrence of hazards as well as the effects thereof. When using properly defined measures and scales, one can treat these methods as objective and repeatable in assessment. An example of a quantitative method is the Events Tree Analysis (ETA), which consists in analysing the consequences resulting from specific events. What follows is the isolation of the triggering event on the basis of which the probable sequences of events are established. In this case, the probability score is the product of the probabilities of all sequences of events. Another example is the Faults Tree Analysis (FTA) method. In contrast to the ETA method, the fault tree in this method is created by starting from the consequences, whereupon they are identified by moving in the direction of the preceding events.

Qualitative methods are based on individual risk estimation using subjective measures. The correctness of inferring from this group of methods is strongly determined by the expertise of the person conducting the assessment. This poses a considerable risk for the application of these methods and contributes to their low repeatability in an assessment done by another person. However, it should be noted that in the case of a person with very extensive expertise on the subject and object of risk assessment, these methods can be very effective as they can contain knowledge resulting

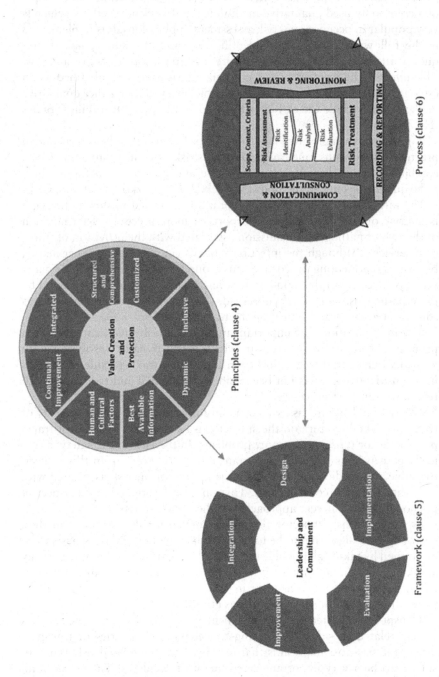

Figure 2.1 Risk management principles, framework and process, based on ISO 31000:2009.

from the expert's experience and association-based deduction. An example of a commonly used qualitative method is the Risk Score method, which is very popular in occupational risk assessment applications. It is implemented in the following steps: hazard identification and assessment, hazard frequency analysis, assessment of exposure time to the hazard factor and possible effects. The result it brings is a quantitative measure obtained as an estimate of the product of the assigned subjective values. Further qualitative methods also include Check List (CHL) and Hazard and Operability Studies (HAZOP).

It is also increasingly often that, both in the literature on the subject and in practical applications, one can come across risk assessment methods which combine selected elements of quantitative and qualitative methods, these to be qualified as mixed methods (Krystek, 2009; Bęczkowski et al., 2013).

The target and subject of the elaborations provided in this monograph is the risk of viral infection in transport, or more precisely, determination of the risk of pathogen transmission associated with the provision of transport services. Although the infection hazards caused, among other actors, by viruses representing the coronavirus group have been imminent for many years, on account of the moderately severe course of the diseases caused by these pathogens, as formerly observed, they have never been perceived as sources of a significant impact on the transport sector.

Risk quantification is an important and continuously investigated research problem. There are many areas in which it still remains unsolved due to individual characteristics. It has been found that, taking epidemic threats into consideration, it has not been sufficiently studied and researched with regard to transport processes.

The risk and hazard assessment is an important task in many areas of transport. The literature on the subject can be reviewed in terms of transport modes or types of transport problems. In the latter case, safety is typically perceived as the most important transport problem. In this respect, the subject of studies and analyses is estimation of the risk associated with accidents and their consequences. This can also be studied in the aspect of methodology or different approaches to the notion of risk.

As for the transport sector, there is no universal risk assessment method or any specific algorithm to be followed, which would enable analysis to be performed by taking all possible factors and hazards into account. Generally speaking, one can find risk analysis methods dedicated to specific hazardous cases, for example, for incidents in road tunnels (the QRA probabilistic method) or for transport of hazardous goods.

Transport-associated risk management in the context of an accident is closely related to safety. According to behavioural theories of transport safety, the basic assumption is that people assess the related risk and consider it to be a very important determinant of accidents. The behavioural theory was confirmed by an example from Sweden. In the autumn of

1967, Sweden switched from left-hand to right-hand traffic organisation. What followed this change was a marked reduction in the traffic fatality rate. About a year and a half later, the accident rate returned to the trend from before the changeover. The perceived risk suddenly became significantly higher than the target level of risk. Road users adjusted their behavioural patterns by choosing much more prudent behaviour alternatives. In a follow-up, the fatal injury rate dropped. After some time, however, drawing from their own experiences, people discovered that roads were not as dangerous as they had thought they were. The level of perceived risk dropped and less often exceeded the target level of risk. Consequently, road users opted for less cautious behaviour alternatives and the fatal injury rate rose again (Wilde, 1994). Numerous other findings can be explained by the risk homeostasis theory, which was primarily developed and validated in the area of road safety.

With this perspective in mind, risk management in transport has evolved. In 1982, Hauer (1982) defined risk as the probability of an accident taking place. The behavioural approach based on the homeostasis theory was presented in a paper by Wilde (1988) published in 1988, while the evolution of this approach was described by Wilde (1998). At the same time, in 1986, Haight (1986) highlighted the consequences of accidents with regard to defining the risk attributable to road transport. Currently, when analysing the accident-associated risk, it is most common that both the probability of an accident taking place and the severity of its consequences are taken into account.

However, some of the research being conducted is also oriented towards other aspects of risk in transport. For example, the fuzzy model of risk assessment has been studied by Polishchuk et al. (2019). These authors compared three methods relevant to an analysis of the comprehensive solutions of environmental start-up projects implemented in the air transport sector. A part of the study by Polishchuk et al. (2019) consisted of using one of the available multi-criteria decision-making methods. Another example of risk assessment vis-à-vis environmental problems is the human health risk assessment of major air pollutants, as presented by Kumar and Mishra (2018). As stated in this paper, the risk of mortality due to air pollution is used to estimate the excess numbers of deaths and illnesses. In the course of their study, Kumar and Mishra (2018) implemented the population attributable risk proportion concept to analyse different input data, such as traffic volumes and vehicular emissions.

Another interesting transport area where risk management was developed is the cyber risk classification framework presented by Sheehan et al. (2019). Cyber risk is defined by the Institute of Risk Management as the risk of financial loss, disruption or damage to the reputation of an organisation from some sort of failure of its information technology systems. The evolution of driverless vehicles and autonomous means of transport evokes many questions, mostly focused on safety. Therefore, hazard and risk assessment in this field is an area which the current research explores. The paper by Sheehan et al. (2019) addresses the Bayesian Network model and the standardised Common Vulnerability Scoring System mechanisms to classify the cyber risk for autonomous vehicles. The paper by Fridstrøm (2020) discusses environmental and sustainability risks attributable to electric vehicles.

Another example of risk assessment in transport is operational risk assessment of offshore transport barges, as presented in Abdussamie et al.(2018). There are numerous methods used for offshore risk assessment which can be categorised as quantitative or qualitative approaches. The analysis by Abdussamie et al. (2018) is based on the hazard identification technique and the risk matrix used for identification of the worst-case scenarios during load-out/float-off operations (Burdzik et al., 2014).

Irrespective of the subject and object of risk management, it can be perceived as a factor decisive of transport-related safety, this being a prerequisite and a basic criterion commonly applied in various spheres, from the design of processes, systems, infrastructure and means of transport to their operation and organisation to their decommissioning or neutralisation. Safety is a fundamental need of every person, social group, organisation and even country. One can also speak of two kinds of safety: internal and external. Stability and a sense of peace are the characteristics of internal safety, while a sense of being unthreatened by forces of nature and other entities are the characteristics of external safety. Threats to safety, in terms of their source of origin, can be divided into two types:

- natural hazards, i.e. consequences of natural forces which can cause disasters,
- civilisational hazards, i.e. human activities which can cause disasters or technical failures.

Threats resulting from pandemics belong to the group of natural hazards, which additionally exert a negative impact on internal safety by creating fear and anxiety in the society caused by changing the manner in which it functions. Consequently, they also affect external safety, which manifests itself in the fear of being infected by potentially contagious persons. The effects of such a perception of safety affect all sectors of transport and transport services, especially in passenger transport.

The safety system implemented in transport is intended to maintain the desired level of safety by shaping solutions which prove to be effective in a specific environment with threats affecting it, which may and do change over time. The most important element of this system is the sphere of risk management, making it possible to analyse and identify: threats, opportunities to reduce the probability of their occurrence, as well as neutralisation and mitigation, once they have been triggered.

The European Guidance on risk assessment proposes an approach based on a number of different steps. This is not the only method used for risk assessment; there is in fact a variety of methodologies designed for achieving the same goal. There is no single *right way* to do a risk assessment, and different approaches can work in different circumstances.

This is particularly noticeable in the transport sector, still lacking a uniform risk management method. However, one can observe individual and separate attempts being made to create foundations for an adequate methodology based on three standard elements: risk analysis, evaluation and assessment; risk elimination; and risk management. Nevertheless, in practical terms, they do not take epidemic threats into account.

To recapitulate the foregoing, up till now (i.e. before the SARS-CoV-2 pandemic), the main aspects addressed in the risk management process in the transport sector have been the potential consequences and the probability of an undesirable event. The assessment of effects consists in estimating losses and other consequences. In freight transport, the effects are mainly defined as non-delivery of cargo or damage to goods, missed deadlines or financial losses. For passenger transport, these are typically understood as damage to or loss of health, including fatalities, lost luggage or delays.

In terms of pandemic threats, the outcome of an epidemic risk assessment should be identification followed by implementation of preventive measures adapted to specific conditions of each mode of transport, intended to minimise the risk of pathogen transmission.

In the case of the SARS-CoV-2 pandemic, effective prevention and control measures have a major impact on the operation of transport enterprises as well as on the safety of transport services. In order for a business to function effectively in this sector, it must develop dedicated procedures and implement epidemic risk management measures.

The preventive measures used to combat the SARS-CoV-2 virus can be classified as either eliminating the threat or minimising and separating the threat from employees, customers and passengers. To this end, specific technical measures, organisational measures, personal protection measures and counter-epidemic measures are used.

The technical measures of collective protection are designed to protect an entire group of people at the same time, including individual persons alone, against harmful and dangerous factors present in the environment. The collective protection measures used when fighting against coronavirus include any kinds of enclosures and partitions separating workers from customers as well as efficient and high-performing ventilation of means of transport. The organisational measures used to contain the spread of the SARS-CoV-2 virus include limiting the number of employees/passengers, remotely controlled and contactless flow of documents and payments, and continuously instructing employees on the applicable safety procedures and rules.

Personal protective equipment designed to keep the entire surface of the human body or the respiratory tract and eyes secured against pathogen transmission into the human organism is also considered very important. These measures are used whenever it is impossible to avoid the hazard at hand, or when it is impossible to sufficiently reduce the threats by other means.

The said counter-epidemic measures aimed at elimination of the SARS-CoV-2 infection risk include increased frequency of cleaning and disinfection of means of transport and workplaces where exposure to the hazardous agents is particularly high. The responsibility for ensuring that these measures are properly implemented as well as for providing the required protective equipment rests with the employer or transport organising institution.

Chapter 3

Matrix of Hazard Assessment in Transport Services in Light of the Threats of the SARS-CoV-2 Pandemic

3.1 DEEP HAZARD IDENTIFICATION (DHI) METHODOLOGY

The problems of risk assessment and management in transport are not new. However, their vast majority involves other problems, for example, safety understood as avoiding accidents involving means of transport, timeliness and elimination of the risk of cargo damage in the case of transport systems and transport organisation. There are very few studies on the risk of infection in transport, and if any can be found, they boil down to modelling the virus spread in the air, which does not allow assessment of the infection risk. Additionally, the second source of infection, which is contact with a contaminated surface, is actually completely ignored.

Therefore, the author of this monograph developed a comprehensive methodology for assessment of epidemic infections risk in transport services, taking into account various hazards and types of virus transmission (droplet and contact surface) based on dedicated scales of hazard evaluation and multi-criteria assessment. The methodology in question is referred to as DHI.

The methodology developed by the author is universal in nature; however, the proposed scales of hazard assessment are dedicated to the epidemic threats of the SARS-CoV-2 coronavirus. The levels of hazard assessment were each time scaled according to the epidemic characteristics of the coronavirus.

While the methodology was being developed, a representative number of different types of transport services were selected. It was assumed that, in order to fully identify the risk factors, transport of both people and goods should be analysed. Passenger transport comprises collective public transport, organised collective transport and individual transport (taxi and car sharing services). The services investigated in the field of goods (freight/cargo) transport are heavy transport and courier parcel delivery. Additionally, specific means and branches of transport were distinguished, and the following transport services were selected for the analysis:

DOI: 10.1201/9781003204732-3

- taxi,
- car sharing,
- mini bus (up to nine passengers),
- coach bus (ordered),
- coach (regular service),
- collective urban transport (bus),
- collective urban transport (tram),
- railway transport (regional),
- railway transport (intercity),
- medical transport (ambulance),
- air transport,
- courier service (parcel locker),
- courier service (d2d),
- food delivery,
- grocery delivery,
- heavy transport (contact),
- heavy transport (no contact).

The methodology developed by the author consists of the following steps (see Figure 3.1):

- developing universal scales to evaluate potential virus transmission mechanisms,
- calculation of the weighting factors to express the mutual significance levels of the assessment criteria,
- mapping transport service processes,
- identification and assessment of potential factors of epidemic threats in the consecutive steps of the transport process,
- determination of a vector (for a single service) or a matrix (for several services) of hazards,
- performing a multi-criteria weighted assessment as a measure of hazard assessment.

3.2 SCALES OF POTENTIAL VIRUS TRANSMISSION MECHANISMS IN TRANSPORTATION SERVICES

The first step in the methodology was to determine all potential virus transmission mechanisms functioning in transport services. In line with the pre-assumed goal, potential mechanisms of the SARS-CoV-2 coronavirus infection were identified as the routes of virus transmission between participants of the transport process by considering transmission by droplets and by contact with contaminated surfaces. Value scaling was performed

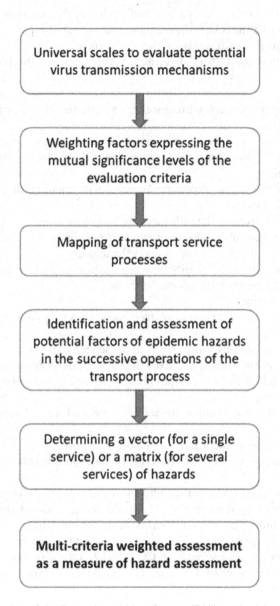

Figure 3.1 Algorithm of the Deep Hazard Identification (DHI) methodology.

according to the current knowledge and epidemic characteristics of the biological hazards of the SARS-CoV-2 pandemic.

Based on an in-depth study of this issue vis-à-vis specific transport services, the following factors determining the infection mechanisms were defined:

- distance in contact with another person for the droplet infection mechanism,
- number of persons per a unit of time who may touch the same surfaces on board means of transport for the surface contact infection mechanism,
- time of the cargo exposure in immediate vicinity of a potentially infected person,
- cargo disinfection methods or cargo isolation time,
- exposure time and number of exposed persons,
- time interval between successive vehicle users,
- exposure time and distance between the operator of the transport process and a potentially infected person,
- transport time,
- distance between seats or free spaces per person in means of transport,
- time between consecutive stops in passenger transport,
- type of air circulation and exchange system in means of transport,
- time and number of persons involved in loading/unloading operations,
- participation of people in activities related to securing cargo for transport,
- type of the document flow system in transport,
- type and form of receipt (delivery) of cargo in transport.

With regard to the first factor (criterion), the current knowledge pertaining to safe distance against the SARS-CoV-2 virus transmission has been reviewed, including the matter of safe distancing measures, such as limiting the density of people in confined spaces, for instance means of transport. When it comes to the spread of COVID-19, safe distance is calculated starting from the level of 1.5–2 m. For purposes of this calculation, one must establish (Sun and Zhai, 2020):

- falling velocity:

$$v_f = \frac{2(\rho - \dot{\rho})}{9\mu} \cdot gr^2 \qquad\qquad (3.1)$$

- falling time:

$$t_f = \frac{H}{v_f} \qquad\qquad (3.2)$$

- horizontal travel distance:

$$d_h = u_0 \times t_f \qquad\qquad (3.3)$$

where:

ρ – particle density (kg/m³),
ρ' – density of flow medium (air, kg/m³),
μ – dynamic viscosity of airflow (Pa·s),
r – radius of particle (m),
g – gravitational acceleration (m/s²),
H – initial height (m),
u_0 – initial velocity (m/s).

What was used to develop the relevant scale was a model that made it possible to study the behaviour of droplets containing the virus (Shafaghi et al., 2020b). In order to adjust the distance to the characteristics of the coronavirus infection, the model uses characteristics of different droplet generation processes, as presented in Xie et al. (2007) and Guerrero et al. (2020) (Table 3.1).

Shafaghi et al. (2020b) discussed model motion of droplets as a function of the time of breathing, sneezing and coughing droplets. Of course, different health organisations recommend different distances. This makes it possible to consider a range of distances (see Figure 3.2).

Based on this knowledge, a scale of hazards related to the distance from another person has been developed against the mechanism of infection by droplets (Table 3.2).

Table 3.1 Parameters of the SARS-CoV-2 droplets for the infection distance calculation

Type of droplet generation	Breathing	Coughing	Sneezing
Initial speed [m/s]	1	10	50
Droplet diameter size	400–900	400–900	400–900
Falling time [s]	4.36	3.11	0.33
Horizontal distance [mm]	432	6,577	3,074

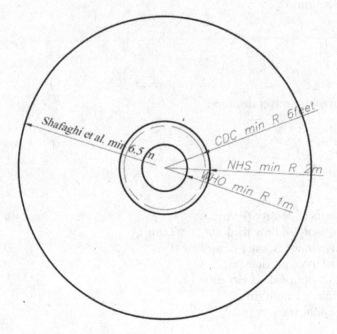

Figure 3.2 Safe distance recommended by different health organisations and in the study by (Shafaghi et al., 2020b).

Table 3.2 Scale of hazards – social distance from another person for the mechanism of infection by droplets

Hazard score	Description
1	Direct contact with another person at a distance of more than 6.5 m.
2	Direct contact with another person at a distance ranging between 3 and 6.5 m.
3	Direct contact with another person at a distance ranging between 1.5 and 3 m.
4	Direct contact with another person at a distance ranging between 0.5 and 1.5 m.
5	Direct contact with another person at a distance of 0.5 m.

Person-to-person transmission of SARS-CoV-2 by droplets is probably the most important factor, but the virus can also be transmitted to a new host via contaminated surfaces. Coronavirus has the capability of persisting on various surfaces for a prolonged time (Mukhra et al., 2020). Therefore, SARS-CoV-2 can be transmitted by indirect contact with the infected person via contaminated surfaces.

Table 3.3 Scale of hazards – threats attributable to touching a contaminated surface in means of transport

Hazard score	Description
1	Direct use of the infrastructure or the vehicle interior by one person within an hour, or disinfection after each user.
2	Direct use of the infrastructure or the vehicle interior by fewer than 10 persons within an hour.
3	Direct use of the infrastructure or the vehicle interior by 10 to 99 persons within an hour.
4	Direct use of the infrastructure or the vehicle interior by 100 to 150 persons within an hour.
5	Direct use of the infrastructure or the vehicle interior by more than 150 persons, or a high probability of contact with an infected person.

Another important aspect of the transport-associated virus transmission mechanism is surface or skin contact. For this purpose, calculations were performed by taking into account the number of people participating in the transport process (passengers or operators) at the same time, in a specific time interval, in specific means of transport. Such assumptions made it possible to estimate the probability of touching the same pieces of equipment on board the vehicle, and thus the probability of virus transmission by surface contact (see Table 3.3).

Another criterion of epidemic risk in transport processes is the time for which the transported cargo (goods) remained in close proximity to a potentially infected person. An average adult's arm's reach was assumed as the range of close distance. In this situation, there was a risk of leaving a biological trace on the cargo, both by droplets and by touch. Specific time intervals were assumed to establish the probability of leaving a biological trace multiple times, which increased in time. What should also be taken into account is that the time for spreading an aerosol over ca. 1.75 m when sneezing takes about 4.5 s, and the aerosol, depending on the particle size, falls to the surface after about 10 min, and it can stay in the air for up to 30 min. Based on studies by dental societies, it was assumed that a significant increase in the risk of infection occurs after 15 min (see Table 3.4).

Another infection risk factor is the time for which the transported cargo has remained without contact with a potential source of infection (human). With regard to this aspect, the time for which the SARS-CoV-2 virus can persist on different surfaces has been analysed (Tables 3.5 and 3.6).

Similarly to the risk of infection by contact with a contaminated surface, specific evaluation criteria were adopted with regard to the time after the lapse of which the vehicle was reused or disinfected (Tables 3.7).

The SARS-CoV-2 virus, like all airborne viruses, is released from an infected individual during coughing, sneezing, talking or even breathing,

Table 3.4 Scale of hazards – time for which cargo (goods) remains in a close distance from a potentially infected person.

Hazard score	Description
1	The cargo has remained in close proximity to a potentially infected person for less than 5 seconds or has been disinfected.
2	The cargo has remained in the vicinity of a potentially infected person for less than 10 min or has been disinfected.
3	The cargo has been kept for 10 to 15 min in close vicinity of a potentially infected person.
4	The cargo has been kept for 15 to 30 min in close vicinity of a potentially infected person.
5	The cargo has remained in the vicinity of a potentially infected person for more than 30 min.

Table 3.5 Time for which the virus persists on contaminated surfaces, based on Mukhra et al. (2020) and (Patients et al., 2020)

Material of surface	Time duration of infection stay
Aerosols	Approximately 3 h
Copper	Not more than 4 h
Cardboard	Not more than 24 h
Plastic, stainless steel	Up to 72 h

Table 3.6 Scale of hazards – time for which cargo in transport remains without contact with a potential source of infection

Hazard score	Description
1	After potential infection, cargo was immediately disinfected.
2	Potentially infected cargo was either isolated from people for more than 72 h or disinfected.
3	After potential infection, cargo was isolated from people for 24 to 48 h.
4	After potential infection, cargo was isolated from people for less than 24 h
5	After potential infection, cargo was not isolated.

and it can persist in the air of a confined space for up to 30 min (Garciá De Abajo et al., 2020). For this reason, another criterion assumed for this purpose was a measure linking the exposure time and the number of persons remaining in the means of transport between disinfection operations (Table 3.8).

When analysing the diverse factors of epidemic threats attributable to transport, not only passengers should be considered, but also employees

Table 3.7 Scale of hazards – time between consecutive uses of means of transport after contact with a potential source of infection

Hazard score	Description
1	Following potential contamination, the vehicle was either isolated for more than 72 h or disinfected after each transport service was completed.
2	Following potential contamination, the vehicle was isolated for 72–48 h and was not disinfected.
3	Following potential contamination, the vehicle was isolated for 48–24 h and was not disinfected.
4	Following potential contamination, the vehicle was isolated for less than 24 h and was not disinfected.
5	Following potential contamination, the vehicle was neither isolated from people nor disinfected.

Table 3.8 Scale of hazards – exposure time and number of persons in the means of transport between disinfection operations

Hazard score	Description
1	Means of transport disinfected after each use.
2	Means of transport used for less than 15 min by fewer than 10 persons, or disinfected.
3	Means of transport used for more than 15 min by more than 10 persons.
4	Means of transport used for more than 30 min by fewer than 10 persons.
5	Means of transport used for more than 15 min by more than 10 persons.

(operators) should be involved in transport services, for both passenger and freight transport. Given the current knowledge (Garciá De Abajo et al., 2020; Shafaghi et al., 2020a) and the pandemic-associated workplace recommendations, the following rating scale has been defined (see Table 3.9).

The time of exposure to potential biological hazards is so important that a decision was made to additionally develop a criterion related to travel time. This criterion proves particularly important with regard to individual transport services, including taxi and car sharing (see Table 3.10).

Social distancing is important for protection against COVID-19, but not only for outdoor spaces but even more important for indoor spaces, including means of transport. Therefore, the next criterion assumed for purposes of this study was the distance between seats and spaces taken by passengers. A 1.5-m distance was assumed as safe. Consequently, the

Table 3.9 Scale of hazards – potential infection depending on worker (operator) exposure time

Hazard score	Description
1	The employee remained in the direct vicinity of a potentially infected person for less than 10 min.
2	The employee remained at a distance of 6.5–2 m from a potentially infected person for 10–15 min.
3	The employee remained at a distance of 6.5–2 m from a potentially infected person for more than 15 min.
4	The employee remained at a distance of less than 2 m from a potentially infected person for 10–15 min.
5	The employee remained at a distance of less than 2 m from a potentially infected person for more than 15 min.

Table 3.10 Scale of hazards – travel (transport) time

Hazard score	Description
1	Transport involves participation of only one driver
2	Less than 10 min
3	From 10 min to 30 min
4	From 30 min to 1 h
5	Over an hour

Table 3.11 Scale of hazards – potential for infection depending on the distance between seats and spaces in vehicles per passenger

Hazard score	Description
1	Transport without passengers – only the driver is onboard the vehicle.
2	Each transport participant has at least 7.1 m^2 of space, and the distance between the seats is not less than 1.5 m.
3	Each transport participant has at least 7.1 m^2 of space, and the distance between the seats is less than 1.5 m.
4	Each transport participant has less than 7.1 m^2 of space, and the distance between the seats is not less than 1.5 m.
5	Each transport participant has less than 7.1 m^2 of space, and the distance between the seats is smaller than 1.5 m

unit measure adopted for this criterion was 1.5 m, regarded as the distance between the available seats and the area of a circle with a radius of 1.5 m, i.e. ca. 7.1 m^2 (see Table 3.11).

As for the analysis of collective urban transport, as well as for courier parcel delivery services, an important factor of epidemic hazard is the dynamics and frequency of passenger exchange (or the potential contact with the courier delivering the parcel). This is due to the probabilities of contact with another infected person (see Table 3.12).

It can be assumed that in the same manner air flow can transfer and deposit infected respiratory droplets/nuclei from infected persons to the mucous membranes of persons standing against the air flow direction (Rule, 2020; Lu et al., 2020; Mouchtouri et al., 2020). Inside means of transport, complex air flows develop on account of the presence of re-circulatory flows driven by ventilation systems and anthropogenic thermally driven flow effects (Shafaghi et al., 2020a). Therefore, the circulation and exchange of air in means of transport were adopted as further factors of the epidemic hazard (see Table 3.13).

With regard to freight transport, the loading and unloading processes are very often overlooked in various analyses. From the point of view of epidemic threats, they are very important because they may involve a direct contact between people or a possibility of contaminating the surface of the cargo. Therefore, in order to comprehensively analyse all hazards, an assessment scale for loading and unloading activities was also developed (see Table 3.14).

Another potential source of infection is the activities related to cargo preparing and securing. There is a risk of contact between operators involved in transport (droplet transmission) or a possibility that a microbial trace is left

Table 3.12 Scale of hazards –frequency and number of stops (delivery points)

Hazard score	Description
1	No stops (delivery points) during the transport service, except for the initial and final stops
2	Time between stops (delivery points) longer than 30 min
3	The time between stops (delivery points) of 10–30 min
4	The time between stops (delivery points) of 5–10 min
5	The time between stops (delivery points) shorter than 5 min.

Table 3.13 Scale of hazards – possible infection depending on air circulation and exchange, as well as air conditioning

Hazard score	Description
1	Air circulation in an open circuit running through HEPA filters
2	Continuous and smooth air exchange inside the vehicle through open-circuit ventilation and opening of windows
3	Air exchange in the vehicle by means of open-circuit ventilation or opening of windows
4	Open circuit air conditioning
5	Air conditioning and air exchange in a closed circuit

Table 3.14 Scale of hazards – potential infection depending on the type of loading and unloading

Hazard score	Description
1	Loading or unloading without contact. The driver remains inside the vehicle cabin and has no contact with the service personnel performing the loading or unloading operations, or with the cargo.
2	Loading or unloading without contact. The driver is responsible for unloading or loading. There is no contact with the service personnel, but there is contact with the cargo.
3	Loading or unloading involving participation of both the driver and the service personnel, which takes less than 10 min.
4	Loading or unloading involving participation of both the driver and the service personnel, which takes 10–30 min.
5	Loading or unloading involving participation of both the driver and the service personnel, which takes more than 30 min.

Table 3.15 Scale of hazards – potential infection conditioned by cargo preparing and securing

Hazard score	Description
1	Cargo is prepared and secured without any contact between the driver and the loader; loading is carried out by one person and the driver has no contact with the cargo.
2	Cargo is prepared and secured without any contact between the driver and the loader; loading is carried out by more than one person and the driver has no contact with the cargo.
3	Cargo is prepared and secured without any contact between the driver and the loader, but the driver has a direct contact with the cargo.
4	Cargo preparing and securing involves participation of both the driver and no more than one operator.
5	Cargo preparing and securing involves participation of both the driver and more than one operator.

on the surface (contact transmission). For this purpose, a dedicated descriptive scale was also developed (see Table 3.15).

What happens very often when analysing the freight transport process is that activities related to the handling of shipping documents are disregarded, while it is precisely during these activities that different people participating in the process may come into a direct contact, or one can contaminate the surface of documents. Therefore, a scale dedicated to this criterion was also prepared (see Table 3.16).

The last criterion was developed to account for the risk of contamination of the parcel or cargo upon the receipt (delivery) (see Table 3.17).

Table 3.16 Scale of hazards – potential infection depending on the document flow
system and driver involvement

Hazard score	Description
1	Contactless flow of documents. The driver remains inside the vehicle cabin and has no contact with a potentially infected person. Fully electronic data exchange.
2	The driver only handles the documents by placing them at a designated point.
3	Direct contact between the driver and a potentially infected person while handing the flow of documents.
4	Direct contact between the driver and a potentially infected person, and signing documents in front of the recipient.
5	Direct contact between the driver and a potentially infected person, and exchange of documents between both parties or signing documents by both parties.

Table 3.17 Scale of hazards – potential infection depending on the delivery point type

Hazard score	Description
1	Contactless delivery to the door or to a point that does not require contact with the infrastructure.
2	Contactless delivery to a point that requires contact with the infrastructure, but without human service.
3	Delivery to a point that requires contact with the infrastructure and the service personnel, while the delivery is collected by one person.
4	Delivery directly to the recipient's hands which involved direct contact with a potentially infected recipient. The delivery is collected by no more than one person.
5	Delivery directly to the recipient's hands which involves direct contact with a potentially infected recipient. The delivery is collected by more than one person.

3.3 ANALYSIS OF THE MUTUAL DOMINATION OF HAZARD FACTORS

Risk assessment is essentially based on a set of factors that strongly influence the eventual outcome or final result. These factors represent grouped sources of hazard, and they affect the risk level differently. Therefore, these hazards should be distinguished according to their impact. This can be considered problematic on account of the multitude of factors that simultaneously affect the final result. For purposes of quantitative assessment of the criteria of impact on the viral infection risk in transport, the Analytic Hierarchy Process (AHP) method was employed (Saaty,

2008). The AHP is a multi-criteria selection method applied when seeking solutions to complex problems that can have multiple objectives which affect decision-making (Librantz et al., 2017). The AHP method makes it possible to relate a decision table and a weight vector based on the pairwise comparison method. The ranking is calculated using a simple additive weighting method.

Decomposition of the problem of the epidemic threats emerging during the SARS-CoV-2 pandemic made it possible to identify the set of criteria described in the previous section. In the next step, a pairwise comparison matrix was created, assumed to function as a matrix of relative importance of individual criteria. A series of in-depth pairwise comparisons was conducted on each level of the hierarchical model. The outcome of comparing two elements from the same level of the hierarchy reflects the preferential dominance between them. In this context, Saaty's (2008) nine-point scale of importance of preferences was used to establish this relationship of dominance (see Table 3.18).

Assuming that the measures of dominance are quantitative, the range between the values of the largest and the smallest measures for each criterion $c = 1, 2, ..., n$ is calculated, and then it is divided into nine intervals, followed by assigning them successive ranks. Comparing the ith variant with the jth variant under the kth criterion, the difference of $b_{ik} - b_{jk}$ is calculated, the absolute value of which indicates the assignment to one of the pre-determined intervals, and thus assignment of an adequate rank.

Finally, matrix $C^k = \left[c_{ij}^{(k)} \right]$, $(i,j = 1,2,...,m,\ k = 1,2,...,n)$ consists of the following elements:

$$c_{ij}^{(k)} = \begin{cases} hazard\ score, & if\ b_{ik}\text{-}b_{jk} \geq 0 \\ 1\ /\ hazard\ score, & if\ b_{ik}\text{-}b_{jk} < 0 \end{cases} \tag{3.4}$$

Table 3.18 Scale of importance of preferences and mutual dominance between criteria C_1 and C_2, based on (Saaty, 2008)

Hazard score	Description
1	Criteria C_1 and C_2 are equally important.
3	Criterion C_1 is slightly more important than C_2.
5	Criterion C_1 is moderately more important than C_2.
7	Criterion C_1 is much more important than C_2.
9	Criterion C_1 is absolutely more important than C_2.
2,4,6,8	Values in-between the above scores of assessment of mutual dominance.

The pairwise comparison process leads to obtaining the following consistent reciprocal matrix (Saaty, 2005):

$$
\begin{array}{cccc}
C_1 & C_2 & \cdots & C_n \\
w_1 & w_2 & \cdots & w_n
\end{array}
$$

$$
\begin{array}{c}
C_1 \\
C_2 \\
\vdots \\
C_n
\end{array}
\begin{bmatrix}
w_1/w_1 & w_1/w_2 & \cdots & w_1/w_n \\
w_2/w_1 & w_2/w_2 & \cdots & w_2/w_n \\
\vdots & \vdots & \vdots & \vdots \\
w_n/w_1 & w_n/w_2 & \cdots & w_n/w_n
\end{bmatrix}
\tag{3.5}
$$

At this stage, a team of transport experts was appointed to individually compare the significance of all criteria following a series of meetings on the SARS-CoV-2 pandemic threats. The results presented in the matrix represent a set of values with the highest numbers obtained for the established group of results.

It can be noted that one can recover the $w = (w_1,...,w_n)$ vector by solving the system of equations defined by:

$$
Cw =
\begin{bmatrix}
w_1/w_1 & w_1/w_2 & \cdots & w_1/w_n \\
w_2/w_1 & w_2/w_2 & \cdots & w_2/w_n \\
\vdots & \vdots & \vdots & \vdots \\
w_n/w_1 & w_n/w_2 & \cdots & w_n/w_n
\end{bmatrix}
\cdot
\begin{bmatrix}
w_1 \\
w_2 \\
\vdots \\
w_n
\end{bmatrix}
= n
\begin{bmatrix}
w_1 \\
w_2 \\
\vdots \\
w_n
\end{bmatrix}
= nw
\tag{3.6}
$$

In order to calculate the value of w, one must solve this homogeneous system of linear equations, i.e. $Cw = nw$. It is an eigenvalue problem because the solution depends on whether or not n is an eigenvalue of the characteristic equation of C. The $C = (c_{ij})$ decision matrix is consistent if $c_{ij}c_{jk} = c_{ik}$, $i,j,k = 1,...,n$ holds among its entries.

In order to interpret and assign relative weights to each criterion, it is necessary to normalise the previous comparison matrix. To this end, the following expression is used:

$$
\hat{w}_{ij}^{(k)} = \frac{c_{ij}^{(k)}}{\sum_{i=1}^{m} c_{ij}^{(k)}}
\tag{3.7}
$$

where m is the criterion number, a sub-criterion or an alternative to be compared.

With reference to the elements of the normalised matrix, individual preference indices (weighting factors) are further determined in accordance with the following formula:

$$w_{ij}^{(k)} = \frac{\sum_{i=1}^{m} \hat{w}_{ij}^{(k)}}{m}$$ (3.8)

The judgements made by those involved in the judging process are evaluated by calculating consistency. First, it is necessary to obtain the maximum value of the eigenvector for each matrix as a coefficient of consistency, given by the following equation:

$$\lambda_{max}^{(k)} = \frac{1}{m} \sum_{i=1}^{m} \frac{c_{ij}^{(k)} \cdot w_{ij}^{(k)}}{w_{ij}^{(k)}}$$ (3.9)

where:

c_{ij} – elements of the C matrix (paired comparisons),
w – weight of criterion,
m – number of criteria.

At this point, it is possible to calculate the consistency index (CI):

$$CI = \frac{|m - \lambda_a|}{m - 1}$$ (3.10)

In terms of the decision-making problem where the AHP method is applied, the consistency of assessments is an important criterion, identical to the transitivity of criteria weights. In order to evaluate the validity, the criteria could be considered consistent, while the value of the calculated consistency ratio should not be greater than 0.1. The compliance rate is determined by the following equation:

$$CR = \frac{CI}{RI(n)}$$ (3.11)

where $RI(n)$ is a fixed value based on the number of criteria, as presented in (Saaty, 2008). If CR is not greater than 0.1, the degree of consistency is satisfactory, but if $CR>0.1$, some serious inconsistencies may have occurred, and the AHP may fail to yield meaningful results.

3.4 PROCESS APPROACH TO IDENTIFICATION OF POTENTIAL FACTORS OF EPIDEMIC HAZARDS IN TRANSPORT SERVICES

The foundation of the contemporary process mapping methods is the flow chart patented by Frank and Lilian Gilbreth in 1921 as a process flow chart. One hypothesised value added through the development and use of the current-state process maps is increased process transparency. In a transparent process, everyone can see and understand the necessary aspects and status of an operation at all times (Klotz et al., 2008). Therefore, process mapping was employed for purposes of the methodology of risk assessment in transport services in light of the epidemic threats during the SARS-CoV-2 pandemic. The purpose of this stage of methodology is identification and assessment of potential factors of the epidemic threats attributable to consecutive operations in a transport process.

Having prepared detailed process maps, one can analyse the potential risk factors (hazards) for each consecutive activity or operation performed by evaluating all the pre-assumed criteria of epidemic risk factors for the SARS-CoV-2 coronavirus infection. For this purpose, one can use the scales of hazard scores presented in Section 3.2.

Due to some discrepancies and the specificity of passenger and freight (cargo) transport, dedicated sets of criteria were proposed, which were divided into two groups. However, in order to fully analyse the imminent hazards, for all transport processes, it was assumed that all criteria assigned to the given group (passenger transport or freight transport) should be assessed.

Such an approach systematises the hazard identification process and makes it possible to compare the results obtained for different transport services in a selected group.

3.5 MULTI-CRITERIA WEIGHTED MATRIX OF HAZARD ASSESSMENT

The main reason for choosing a multi-criteria approach for the methodology developed by the author is the multitude of different perspectives, targets, criteria or preferences that are prioritised by each stakeholder (Hopfe et al., 2013).

In the first stage, the process should be analysed in terms of the defined criteria determining the epidemic hazards in transport services by tracking process maps (section 3.4), followed by their assessment in accordance with the scales developed (section 3.2). As a result of the foregoing, one obtains a multivalent vector of the hazard state of a transport service, which is standardised in terms of elementary values and size, making it quantitatively comparable with other services. The transport service epidemic hazard state vector is defined as a column vector:

$$h = \begin{bmatrix} h_{c_1} \\ h_{c_2} \\ \vdots \\ h_{c_n} \end{bmatrix} \tag{3.12}$$

Due to the differences in the impact of various hazard factors on the immediate threats of the SARS-CoV-2 coronavirus infection, the state vector thus determined should be adjusted with appropriate weighting factors for each of the criteria (section 3.3). This is expressed in the following equation:

$$h \cdot w \overset{\text{def}}{=} \begin{bmatrix} h_{c_1} & \cdot & w_1 \\ h_{c_2} & \cdot & w_2 \\ \vdots & \ddots & \vdots \\ h_{c_n} & \cdot & w_n \end{bmatrix} \tag{3.13}$$

Consequently, it is possible to quantify hazards for the chosen transport service and express them with a specific value as a scalar product:

$$(h,w) = h^T w = w^T h \overset{\text{def}}{=} \sum_{i=1}^{n} h_i w_i = h_{ti} \tag{3.14}$$

This estimator is referred to as the DHI index. Its values are consistent with the range of criteria evaluation scales. In the case subject to analysis, these range between 1 and 5 for the entire sector of transport services. The DHI index range, separate for passenger and freight transport, assumes values consistent with the adjusted weights of the sum of group criteria.

By repeating these calculations for consecutive transport services while maintaining all the assumptions of the methodology in question, one will obtain the matrix of hazard assessment for transport services in light of the threads of the SARS-CoV-2 pandemic according to the following equation:

$$H\left(c_{ij}\right) = \begin{bmatrix} h_{1,c_1} \cdot w_1 & h_{2c_1} \cdot w_1 & \cdots & h_{mc_1} \cdot w_1 \\ h_{1c_2} \cdot w_2 & h_{2c_2} \cdot w_2 & \cdots & h_{mc_2} \cdot w_2 \\ \vdots & \vdots & \vdots & \vdots \\ h_{1c_n} \cdot w_n & h_{2c_n} \cdot w_n & \cdots & h_{mc_n} \cdot w_n \end{bmatrix} = h_t \tag{3.15}$$

The matrix of hazard assessment for transport services in light of the threats of the SARS-CoV-2 pandemic makes it possible to determine a collective table of hazard factors for a selected group of transport services. It enables identification of the dominant hazard sources and allows for comparison of the chosen services against the context of the epidemic threats. This may provide the grounds for making decisions regarding the selection of transport services or indicating a hierarchy of goals in the context of minimising or eliminating the relevant risk factors.

3.6 CASE STUDIES

3.6.1 Weighting Factors Expressing Mutual Significance Levels of Assessment Criteria

The aspect of mutual dominance of hazard factors has been analysed by following the methodology discussed in section 3.1. The scales described in section 3.2 have been used to assess each criterion.

The results presented below are values representative of the assessment, dominating among individual assessments done by transport experts. The persons participating in the dominance analysis represent a group of people involved in a wider project implemented in the field of epidemic risk identification in transport services. Therefore, it should be assumed that their knowledge and awareness of the subject is very up-to-date and extensive.

Additionally, Table 3.19 contains the computed total values expressing the dominance of individual criteria and the percentage share among all the criteria. This allows for the criteria to be classified according to their significance.

Using the modified AHP method (section 3.3), the normalised matrix of weighting factors provided in Table 3.20 has been developed to represent the mutual significance levels of the evaluation criteria.

Consequently, the following weighting factors have been identified for all the criteria adopted (see Table 3.21):

The matrix thus obtained is consistent since its maximum eigenvalue is $\lambda_{max}=16.8656$, while its consistency index $CI=0.133257$ and its consistency ratio $CR=0.0838095$, which is a satisfactory value, being much smaller than

Table 3.19 Final report from an expert study on mutual dominance between criteria (pairwise matrix)

Pairwise comparison matrix A\B	social distance (droplets)	touching a contaminated surface	loading time	isolation time (cargo)	time between use cases	exposure time and number of persons	operator exposure time	transport time	distance between seats	number of stops	air circulation	type of loading opeation	securing the cargo	document flow	type of delivery point	total score	max possible score = 135
social distance (droplets)	1	3	9	7	7	1	2	3	2	7	3	9	7	7	7	75,00	55,56%[a]
touching a contaminated surface	1/3	1	7	5	7	1/7	1/5	1/2	1	3	2	7	5	5	3	47,18	34,95%
loading time	1/9	1/7	1	1/3	1/3	1/9	1/7	1/5	1/6	1/5	1/6	2	1/2	3	1/3	8,74	6,48%
isolation time (cargo)	1/7	1/5	3	1	1	1/9	1/7	1/7	1/5	1/3	1/3	5	5	5	2	23,61	17,49%
time between use cases	1/7	1/7	3	1	1	1/9	1/5	1	1/5	1/3	1/3	2	2	1	1	13,86	10,27%
exposure time and number of persons	1	7	9	9	9	1	3	3	3	6	3	9	9	7	5	84,00	62,22%
operator exposure time	1/2	5	7	7	5	1/3	1	2	3	3	3	7	9	5	7	64,83	48,02%
transport time	1/3	2	5	7	1	1/3	1/2	1	1/2	5	7	7	7	9	7	59,67	44,20%
distance between seats	1/2	1	6	5	5	1/3	1/3	1/2	1	5	2	7	7	7	7	56,17	41,60%
number of stops	1/7	1/3	5	3	3	1/6	1/3	1/5	1/5	1	1/5	5	3	3	2	26,65	19,74%
air circulation	1/3	1/2	6	3	3	1/3	1/3	1/7	1/2	5	1	7	5	5	5	42,20	31,26%
type of loading opeation	1/9	1/7	1/2	1/5	1/2	1/9	1/7	1/7	1/7	1/5	1/7	1	1	1/3	1/2	5,84	4,32%
securing the cargo	1/7	1/5	2	1/5	1/2	1/9	1/9	1/7	1/7	1/3	1/5	1	1	1	1/2	7,39	5,47%
document flow	1/7	1/5	1/3	1/5	1	1/7	1/5	1/9	1/7	1/3	1/5	3	1	1	1	9,34	6,92%
type of delivery point	1/7	1/3	3	1/2	1	1/5	1/7	1/7	1/7	1/2	1/5	2	2	1	1	12,55	9,30%

Note
[a] Italic values represents the calculation (not data).

Table 3.20 Matrix of weighting factors expressing the mutual significance levels of the evaluation criteria

Pairwise comparison matrix A\B	social distance (droplets)	touching a contaminated surface	loading time	isolation time (cargo)	time between use cases	exposure time and number of persons	operator exposure time	transport time	distance between seats	number of stops	air circulation	type of loading operation	securing the cargo	document flow	type of delivery point	average
social distance (droplets)	0,20	0,14	0,13	0,14	0,13	0,22	0,23	0,23	0,16	0,19	0,14	0,13	0,10	0,11	0,16	**0,16**
touching a contaminated surface	0,07	0,05	0,10	0,10	0,13	0,03	0,02	0,04	0,08	0,08	0,10	0,10	0,07	0,08	0,07	**0,07**
loading time	0,02	0,01	0,01	0,01	0,01	0,02	0,02	0,02	0,01	0,01	0,01	0,03	0,01	0,05	0,01	**0,02**
isolation time (cargo)	0,03	0,01	0,04	0,02	0,02	0,02	0,02	0,01	0,02	0,01	0,02	0,07	0,07	0,08	0,05	**0,03**
time between use cases	0,03	0,01	0,04	0,02	0,02	0,02	0,02	0,02	0,02	0,01	0,01	0,03	0,03	0,05	0,01	**0,02**
exposure time and number of persons	0,20	0,33	0,13	0,18	0,17	0,22	0,34	0,23	0,24	0,16	0,14	0,13	0,13	0,11	0,11	**0,19**
operator exposure time	0,10	0,24	0,10	0,14	0,09	0,07	0,11	0,15	0,24	0,08	0,014	0,10	0,13	0,08	0,16	**0,13**
transport time	0,07	0,09	0,07	0,14	0,09	0,07	0,06	0,08	0,04	0,08	0,24	0,10	0,13	0,15	0,11	**0,10**
distance between seats	0,10	0,05	0,09	0,10	0,09	0,07	0,04	0,15	0,08	0,19	0,10	0,10	0,10	0,11	0,11	**0,10**
number of stops	0,03	0,02	0,07	0,06	0,06	0,04	0,04	0,03	0,01	0,03	0,01	0,07	0,04	0,05	0,05	**0,04**
air circulation	0,07	0,02	0,09	0,06	0,09	0,07	0,04	0,02	0,04	0,13	0,05	0,10	0,07	0,08	0,07	**0,07**
type of loading operation	0,02	0,01	0,01	0,00	0,01	0,02	0,02	0,01	0,01	0,01	0,01	0,01	0,01	0,01	0,02	**0,01**
securing the cargo	0,03	0,01	0,03	0,00	0,01	0,02	0,01	0,01	0,01	0,01	0,01	0,01	0,01	0,01	0,02	**0,01**
document flow	0,03	0,01	0,00	0,00	0,01	0,03	0,02	0,01	0,01	0,01	0,01	0,03	0,04	0,02	0,02	**0,02**
type of delivery point	0,03	0,02	0,04	0,01	0,06	0,04	0,02	0,02	0,02	0,01	0,02	0,01	0,01	0,02	0,02	**0,02**
Sum:	1,00	1,00	1,00	1,00	1,00	1,00	1,00	1,00	1,00	1,00	1,00	1,00	1,00	1,00	1,00	1,00

Table 3.21 Weighting factors of the DHI methodology criteria

Criterion number	Criterion	Weighting factors
1	social distance (droplets)	0,16
2	touching a contaminated surface	0,07
3	loading time	0,02
4	isolation time (cargo)	0,03
5	time between use cases	0,02
6	exposure time and number of persons	0,19
7	operator exposure time	0,13
8	transport time	0,10
9	distance between seats	0,10
10	number of stops	0,04
11	air circulation	0,07
12	type of loading operation	0,01
13	securing the cargo	0,01
14	document flow	0,02
15	type of delivery point	0,02
	SUM:	1,00

0.1. Consequently, the weighting factors thus calculated should be regarded as adequate.

3.6.2 Process Approach to Identification of Potential Factors of the Epidemic Threats Attributable to Transport Services

As a part of the research, a detailed analysis of the sources of hazard was conducted using the methodology intended for mapping the processes of all transport services, as introduced in Section 3.4. The monograph provides examples of process maps and identification of hazard factors for three different transport services, dividing them into main groups corresponding to passenger and freight (cargo) transport. The hazard factors were identified by evaluating all 15 criteria according to the scales previously designed (scores ranging between 1 and 5), analysing all activities and operations in the process map, one by one. Such an approach guarantees universality and comparability of assessments for various transport services, and represents a comprehensive concept of an in-depth step-by-step analysis.

Process mapping is required for the purpose of the DHI methodology, which means that it should only focus on all those activities or operations that involve the risk of virus transmission. What follows is a discussion on the three case studies provided below.

3.6.3 Case Study of Collective Urban Transport

First, it should be noted that in the case of collective urban transport, one deals with randomness in terms of participation and flow of passengers, which increases the probability that there are persons infected with the virus (especially the asymptomatic ones) among those involved in the service. Additionally, an assessment of the scale of the risk effects should also consider the inability to identify the chain of infections in order that the persons who may continue to transmit the virus can be isolated post factum.

Figure 3.3 illustrates the map of transport services analysed with respect to the potential occurrence of contact (either interpersonal or with a contaminated surface).

Table 3.22 summarises the identification and assessment of the possibility of epidemic hazard according to the pre-assumed criteria which affect the mechanisms of infection (virus transmission) in transport services.

3.6.4 Case Study of Car Sharing

Figure 3.4 provides a map of the relevant transport service, drawn up by considering the possibility of contact (interpersonal or with a surface).

The map of this process shows that there are just one or two direct contact possibilities (or even none), but there are still infection hazards due to surface contact transmission. The identification and assessment of the potential epidemic hazard attributable to the car sharing services is summarised in Table 3.23.

3.6.5 Case Study of Courier Parcel Delivery Services

Figure 3.5 represents a map of the courier transport service, drawn up by considering the possibility of contact (interpersonal or with a surface).

Given the significant differences in the potential coronavirus infection hazards depending on the delivery type (personal collection vs. parcel locker), separate analyses should be performed. In the example described below, a general variant was adopted, emphasising the differences in the scoring of hazards. Table 3.24 summarises the identification and assessment of the potential epidemic hazard related to courier parcel delivery services.

The foregoing case studies show how to proceed according to the DHI method, and how to perform the relevant analysis by deductive reasoning in order to determine the score of epidemic hazards according to consecutive criteria, without considering the relevance and significance of these criteria.

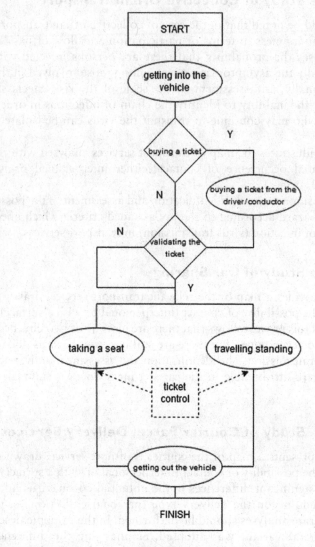

Figure 3.3 Collective urban transport process mapping in terms of the DHI methodology.

Table 3.22 Assessment of epidemic hazards according to the DHI methodology criteria – collective urban transport

Criterion	Description	Hazard score
Social distance (droplets)	Passengers engage in conversations with one another, hence the possibility of coughing and sneezing. The distance between passengers can range between 0.5 and 1.5 m. Additionally, there are shared transport corridors and entrance doors in which people crowd for a short time.	4
Touching a contaminated surface	Contamination of vehicle components such as handles, handrails, seats and other elements inside the vehicle within the passenger's reach. Direct contact during ticket control. Assuming that a bus journey takes about 20 min, while the average number of available places is 33 (typically 110 standing places and seats) given the restrictions imposed (30% of vehicle carrying capacity), hence the possibility that 99 persons can use the given vehicle over an hour.	3
Exposure time and number of persons	Once the service has been performed, the vehicle is not cleaned by the transport company's staff. The vehicle-associated exposure is longer than 30 min, and it is operated by more than 10 people during this period.	5
Time between use cases	The vehicle features many plastic elements on which the virus can persist for the longest time (up to 72 h), thus posing a threat. After the service, the vehicle is not cleaned by the transport company's staff, nor is it subjected to isolation.	5
Operator exposure time	The operator (driver) remains in the presence of a potential hazard for more than 15 min at a distance of more than 2 m.	3
Transport time	Assuming that regular transport services are typically delivered over short routes (in-city connections), the duration of such a service can be assumed between 10 and 30 min.	3
Distance between seats	The space available in buses is approximately 47.8 m^2. Given that 7.1 m^2 was assumed as a safe space, only six persons could safely travel on board of such a bus. Additionally, the distance between seats is less than 1.5 m.	5
Number of stops	The stops in transport services are frequent, and the time interval between them is often shorter than 5 min.	5
Air circulation	In older vehicles, it is possible to exchange the air in an open circuit by opening a window or switching the air-conditioning system on. However, the newer ones feature an air-conditioned closed air circulation system. Therefore, an average value ranging between 3 and 5 was adopted.	4
Total score:		**37**

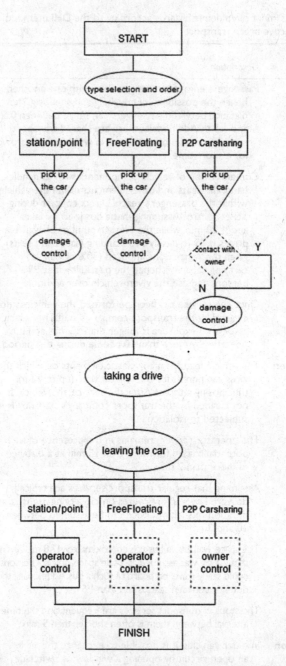

Figure 3.4 Car sharing process mapping in terms of the DHI methodology.

Table 3.23 Assessment of epidemic hazards according to the DHI methodology criteria – car sharing

Criterion	Description	Hazard score
Social distance (droplets)	There is often only one person on board a vehicle; if there are more, they are typically familiar with each other (mutually aware of the other's health condition).	1
Touching a contaminated surface	Potential contamination of vehicle components – exterior door handles, interior door handles, seats, seat belts and other components inside the vehicle within easy reach. It is assumed that within an hour the vehicle is only used by the driver, which, given the average use time of 30 min, results in an exchange of two persons per hour. The vehicle is not cleaned after each use.	2
Exposure time and number of persons	The vehicle is not cleaned after each use. Hence, the assumption that the vehicle's exposure is over 30 min, and during that time it is operated by less than 10 persons.	4
Time between use cases	The car features many plastic elements on which the virus can persist for the longest (up to 72 h), thus posing a threat. The vehicle is not cleaned after each use. Within 72 h, on average, up to 120 persons can use the car.	5
Operator exposure time	The operator has no contact with the customer.	1
Transport time	Transport takes place with the participation of only one driver.	1
Distance between seats	The square area of passenger cars is approximately 2.5–3.7 m², and the distance between the seats is less than 1.5 m. However, it was assumed that the driver is alone on board the vehicle.	1
Number of stops	There are no stops involved in the service, and the transport takes place directly between the start point and the end point.	1
Air circulation	In passenger vehicles, it is possible to exchange air in an open circuit, both by opening windows and by switching the ventilation system on, thus ensuring smooth air exchange.	2
Total score:		18

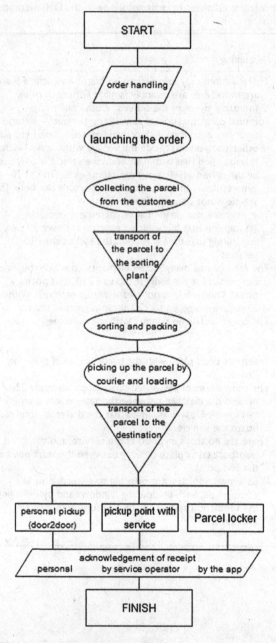

Figure 3.5 Courier parcel delivery service process mapping in terms of the DHI methodology.

Table 3.24 Assessment of epidemic hazards according to the DHI methodology criteria – courier parcel delivery services

Criterion	Description	Hazard score
Social distance (droplets)	There may be direct contact between employees of the courier company, but currently the contact between the courier and the customer has been virtually eliminated. This is only the case of direct parcel collection, which is estimated at 10–15% in the current situation, which still represents a safe contact assuming that a protective mask is used (for personal delivery, the score can even be 5).	1
Touching a contaminated surface	Several employees (up to 10) at the reloading point have direct contact with the shipment. There is contact between the cargo and vehicle interior elements, including the cargo area. The vehicle is usually used by one employee within an hour's time or even throughout a whole day (score 2). In personal delivery, there is a close contact with the customer when the shipment is sent/received (score 4).	2
Loading time	From the moment of collection from the sender, shipments are in contact with the courier upon receipt, delivery to the reloading point, picking up from the reloading point and delivery to the collection point. Assuming that each of these activities takes up to 2 min on average (picking up, putting away and scanning the barcode), the exposure of the shipments takes less than 10 min (for personal delivery, this can come to 10–15 min – score 3)	2
Isolation time (cargo)	The time between the receipt of goods from the transhipment point to their release to the collection point is usually no more than 12 h. In the case of parcel lockers, the delivery time is usually 48 h (score 3). Therefore, it is possible to isolate the goods from harmful factors, but it depends on the customer's will. Direct collection is immediate (score 5).	4
Time between use cases	The car features many plastic elements on which the virus can persist for the longest time (up to 72 h), thus posing a threat. After the entire workday, the vehicle is handed over to another employee or to the one who has been using the vehicle on that day. It is not subject to disinfection and isolation after each user has stopped using it.	5
Operator exposure time	The courier may have a short-term contact with other employees when shipments are released to the reloading point and picked up from the reloading point, or with customers in the event of personal collection. Assuming that each of these activities takes up to 2 min on average (picking up, putting away, scanning the barcode, and handing over the parcel), the employee's total exposure ranges from 10 min to 30 min.	5

(continued)

Table 3.24 Cont.

Criterion	Description	Hazard score
Number of stops	In the case of non-contact delivery (parcel lockers), the number of stops does not matter as there is no risk of the courier becoming infected (score 1). In direct delivery, this number can increase to even a dozen persons (every 30 min), but this involves a very direct short contact, and the required preventive measures (masks) are assumed to be in use (score 3).	2
Air circulation	In vehicles, it is possible to exchange air in an open circuit system, using ventilation and by opening windows.	2
Type of loading operation	The parcel is sent by the customer at a parcel locker without any interpersonal contact. The courier picks up and delivers the package on its own, again without contact. There is no contact with the service personnel/customer, but there is a contact with the cargo (score 2). In the case of personal delivery, the parcel sending by the customer involves some contact. Couriers pick up and deliver packages themselves. There is a contact with the customer and the shipments (score 3).	2
Securing the cargo	Couriers collect the goods from the parcel locker and secure them on the vehicle by themselves. At the sorting plant, the goods are also secured (packed) by one employee.	3
Document flow	A majority of courier services are handled using fully electronic data interchange (score 1). However, when goods are home delivered, documents are signed by electronic means (score 4).	1
Type of delivery point	Contactless delivery entails using parcel lockers, which eliminates any contact between couriers and any other persons, but they contact with the infrastructure of the given facility (score 2). Home delivery involves a contact. The driver has a direct contact with the recipient, but the pickup is performed by one person (score 4).	2
Total score:		**29**

3.6.6 Multi-Criteria Weighted Hazard Assessment

The tables provided in the previous section make it possible to determine a multivalued vector of the epidemic hazard state of a transport service. However, due to the differences in terms of the effect on the immediate threats of the SARS-CoV-2 coronavirus infection from various hazard factors, the state vector thus determined should be adjusted with appropriate weighting factors. Additionally, on account of the specificity of passenger and freight (cargo) transport, the hazard identification criteria were also selectively grouped, and, therefore, the comparison was each time made separately for two groups of transport services (passenger transport and freight transport).

Table 3.25 Assessment of the DHI index, provided as a total weighted value of hazard – passenger transport

Hazard	Weighting factors	Collective urban transport – score	Collective urban transport – weighting score	Car sharing – score	Car sharing – weighting score
Social distance (droplets)	0.16	4	0.65	1	0.16
Touching a contaminated surface	0.07	3	0.22	2	0.15
Exposure time and number of persons	0.19	5	0.95	4	0.76
Time between use cases	0.02	5	0.11	5	0.11
Operator exposure time	0.13	3	0.39	1	0.13
Transport time	0.10	3	0.31	1	0.10
Distance between seats	0.10	5	0.50	1	0.10
Number of stops	0.04	5	0.20	1	0.04
Air circulation	0.07	4	0.27	2	0.13
TOTAL:		**37**	**3.59**	**18.00**	**1.68**

Table 3.26 Assessment of the DHI index, as a total weighted value of hazard – courier parcel delivery services

Hazard	Weighting factors	Courier service (parcel locker) – score	Courier service (parcel locker) – weighting score	Courier service (d2d)	Courier service (d2d) – weighting score
Social distance (droplets)	0.16	1	0.16	5	0.81
Touching a contaminated surface	0.07	2	0.15	4	0.30
Loading time	0.02	2	0.03	3	0.05
Isolation time (cargo)	0.03	3	0.10	5	0.16
Time between use cases	0.02	5	0.11	3	0.07
Operator exposure time	0.13	5	0.65	5	0.65
Number of stops	0.04	1	0.04	3	0.12
Air circulation	0.07	2	0.13	2	0.13
Type of loading operation	0.01	2	0.02	3	0.04
Securing the cargo	0.01	3	0.04	3	0.04
Document flow	0.02	1	0.02	4	0.07
Type of delivery point	0.02	2	0.05	4	0.09
TOTAL:		**29**	**1.50**	**44**	**2.52**

The results of the associated transformations are provided in the Tables 3.25 and 3.26.

As a result of the multi-criteria weighted hazard assessment (DHI index) with reference to the above examples of collective urban passenger transport, the weighted score of the DHI index was determined at 3.59, while for car sharing, the DHI index was 1.68. With regard to the examples of cargo transport by courier services (parcel locker), the weighted score of the DHI index was determined at 1.50, while for the door to door (d2d) courier services, the DHI index came to 2.52. The risk levels established on the basis of these values have been interpreted in next chapter.

3.7 DISCUSSION

In order to emphasise the significance of the results obtained under the afore-mentioned analyses, the following matrix of hazard assessment addressing a large group of transport services has been provided further on.

The methodology developed by the author for purposes of the assessment of the epidemic hazard of viral infection using the example of the SARS-CoV-2 coronavirus pandemic, referred to as DHI, enables quantitative assessment of hazards based on the vector of the state of epidemic hazards.

With reference to the data sets and process maps developed for the chosen group of transport services, it is possible to determine the matrix of hazard assessment. The author recommends making a selective choice of assessment criteria depending on the transport service type. In the most general terms, it is also recommended that transport services should be divided into passenger and freight (cargo) transport. Given the reduced number of the criteria assumed in the analysis, the final weighted estimator becomes even more representative. As part of the discussion, the author has assessed 17 groups of transport services, including 11 passenger transport and 6 freight transport services.

The scoring results are provided in Table 3.27.

The final evaluation has been adjusted with the weighting factors of the assumed criteria, consequently obtaining a multi-criteria weighted matrix of hazard assessment for passenger transport services (Table 3.28).

This enables a quantitative comparison of the value of epidemic hazard attributable to passenger transport services. Based on the preceding analyses, the highest score of epidemic hazard has been established for regular coach services (DHI = 3.98), while the second highest score has been obtained for mini bus transport services (DHI = 3.93). By far the lowest value has been determined for car sharing services (DHI = 1.68). Moreover, this method makes it possible to compare the percentage values in the passenger transport group only, or against the entire transport sector, thus obtaining overall share values, without any breakdown into service groups. This distribution is shown in Figure 3.6.

An analysis of the selected representative freight transport services was performed in a similar manner. Summaries of the hazard assessments and the values adjusted by weighting factors are provided Tables 3.29 and 3.30.

Based on the aforementioned analyses, the highest value of epidemic hazard has been found to represent the door-to-door courier parcel delivery

Table 3.27 Multi-criteria assessment of the hazard matrix for passenger transport services

Hazard	Weighting factors	taxi	Car sharing	Mini bus (up tp 9 passengers)	Coach bus (ordered)	Coach bus (regular service)	Collective urban transport (bus)	Collective urban transport (tram)	Railway transport (regional)	Railway transport (intercity)	Medical transport (ambulance)	Air transport
Social distance (droplets)	0,16	5	1	5	5	5	4	4	4	5	5	5
Touching a contaminated surface	0,07	2	2	4	3	3	3	3	3	3	5	5
Exposure time and number of persons	0,19	4	4	4	5	5	5	5	5	4	3	5
time between use cases	0,02	5	5	4	1	3	5	5	5	5	1	1
Operator exposure time	0,13	5	1	5	5	5	3	3	2	2	5	2
Transport time	0,10	3	1	5	5	5	3	3	4	5	3	5
Distance between seats	0,10	5	1	5	5	5	5	5	5	5	5	5
Number of stops	0,04	1	1	3	1	2	5	5	4	2	1	1
Air circulation	0,07	2	2	3	3	3	4	4	3	3	3	1
Sum:		32	18	38	33	36	37	37	35	34	31	30

Table 3.28 Multi-criteria weighted matrix of hazard assessment for passenger transport services

Hazard	Weighting factors	Taxi	Car sharing	Mini bus (up to 9 passengers)	Coach bus (ordered)	Coach bus (regular service)	Collective urban transport (bus)	Collective urban transport (tram)	Railway transport (regional)	Railway transport (intercity)	Medical transport (ambulance)	Air transport
Social distance (droplets)	0,16	0,81	0,16	0,81	0,81	0,81	0,65	0,65	0,65	0,81	0,81	0,81
Touching a contaminated surface	0,07	0,15	0,15	0,30	0,22	0,22	0,22	0,22	0,22	0,22	0,37	0,37
Exposure time and number of persons	0,19	0,76	0,76	0,76	0,95	0,95	0,95	0,95	0,95	0,76	0,57	0,95
Time between use cases	0,02	0,11	0,11	0,09	0,02	0,07	0,11	0,11	0,11	0,11	0,02	0,02
operator exposure time	0,13	0,65	0,13	0,65	0,65	0,65	0,39	0,39	0,26	0,26	0,65	0,26
Transport time	0,10	0,31	0,10	0,51	0,51	0,51	0,31	0,31	0,41	0,51	0,31	0,51
Distance Between seats	0,10	0,50	0,10	0,50	0,50	0,50	0,50	0,50	0,50	0,50	0,50	0,50
Number of stops	0,04	0,04	0,04	0,12	0,04	0,08	0,20	0,20	0,16	0,08	0,04	0,04
Air circulation	0,07	0,13	0,13	0,20	0,20	0,20	0,27	0,27	0,20	0,20	0,20	0,07
Sum:		3,45	1,68	3,93	3,90	3,98	3,59	3,59	3,45	3,45	3,47	3,52
% from passenger transport:		78,01%	38,05%	88,80%	88,11%	90,00%	81,04%	81,04%	77,99%	77,88%	78,33%	79,63%
% from all transport services		69,02%	33,67%	78,58%	77,97%	79,64%	71,71%	71,71%	69,01%	68,91%	69,31%	70,46%

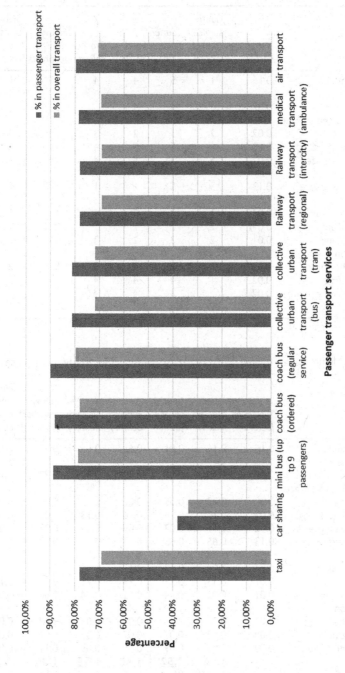

Figure 3.6 Percentage DHI indices from the epidemic hazard assessment for passenger transport services.

Table 3.29 Multi-criteria assessment of the hazard matrix for freight transport services

Hazard	Weighting factors	Courier service (parcel locker)	Courier service (d2d)	Food delivery	Grocery delivery	Heavy transport (contact)	Heavy transport (no contact)
Social distance (droplets)	0.16	1	5	4	4	3	1
Touching a contaminated surface	0.07	2	4	4	5	3	2
Loading time	0.02	2	3	2	3	2	2
Isolation time (cargo)	0.03	3	5	5	4	2	2
Time between use cases	0.02	5	3	4	4	1	1
Operator exposure time	0.13	5	5	1	1	1	1
Number of stops	0.04	1	3	3	4	1	1
Air circulation	0.07	2	2	2	2	2	2
Type of loading operation	0.01	2	3	2	3	5	1
Securing the cargo	0.01	3	3	4	3	5	2
document flow	0.02	1	4	4	4	5	5
Type of delivery point	0.02	2	4	4	4	5	1
Total:		**29**	**44**	**39**	**41**	**35**	**21**

Table 3.30 Multi-criteria weighted matrix of hazard assessment for freight transport services

Hazard	Weighting factors	Courier service (parcel locker)	Courier service (d2d)	Food delivery	Grocery delivery	Heavy transport (contact)	Heavy transport (no contact)
Social distance (droplets)	0.16	0.16	0.81	0.65	0.65	0.48	0,16
Touching a contaminated surface	0.07	0.15	0.30	0.30	0.37	0.22	0,15
Loading time	0.02	0.03	0.05	0.03	0.05	0.03	0,03
Isolation time (cargo)	0.03	0.10	0.16	0.16	0.13	0.06	0,06
Time between use cases	0.02	0.11	0.07	0.09	0.09	0.02	0,02
Operator exposure time	0.13	0.65	0.65	0.13	0.13	0.13	0,13
Number of stops	0.04	0.04	0.12	0.12	0.16	0.04	0,04
Air circulation	0.07	0.13	0.13	0.13	0.13	0.13	0,13
Type of loading operation	0.01	0.02	0.04	0.02	0.04	0.06	0,01
Securing the cargo	0.01	0.04	0.04	0.06	0.04	0.07	0,03
Document flow	0.02	0.02	0.07	0.07	0.07	0.09	0,09
Type of delivery point	0.02	0.05	0.09	0.09	0.09	0.11	0,02
total:		**1.50**	**2.52**	**1.85**	**1.95**	**1.46**	**0.88**
% share of cargo transport		48.42%	81.25%	59.55%	62.62%	47.10%	28.38%
% share of all transport services		30.09%	50.48%	37.00%	38.91%	29.27%	17.64%

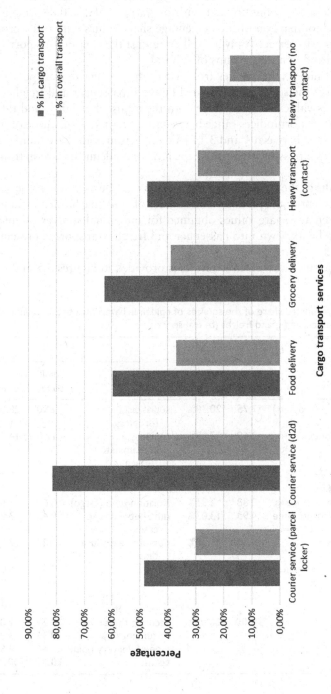

Figure 3.7 Percentage DHI indices from the epidemic hazard assessment for freight transport services.

services (DHI = 2.52). The lowest value is definitely the one established for heavy transport without contact with operators (DHI = 0.88). Figure 3.7 illustrates a comparison of the percentage share values within the group of freight transport services only as well as against the overall transport sector, without breakdown into groups of services.

The DHI index takes values from 1 to 5 for the entire transport service sector. Where the services are divided between passenger and freight transport, it takes values in accordance with the adjusted weights, and thus the passenger transport indices range between 1 and 4.44, while those of freight transport range between 1 and 3.11. A comparison with these limited range values makes it possible to estimate the level of epidemic hazard in transport service.

The results of the hazard assessment matrix can be used otherwise as well, namely, to identify the predominant sources of epidemic hazard. A summary of the percentage share values obtained for individual sources of epidemic hazard in a breakdown into passenger and freight transport is presented in Table 3.31.

A graphic summary of these results is provided in Figures 3.8 and 3.9.

Table 3.31 Percentage share of the sources of epidemic hazard in a breakdown into passenger (a) and freight (b) transport

a)			b)		
hazard	Total score	percentage	hazard	Total score	percentage
social distance (droplets)	7.75	20.38%	social distance (droplets)	2.90	28.56%
Touching a contaminated surface	2.69	7.09%	touching a contaminated surface	1.50	14.72%
Exposure time and number of persons	9.28	24.41%	loading time	0.22	2.12%
Time between use cases	0.88	2.31%	isolation time (cargo)	0.68	6.67%
Operator exposure time	4.95	13.03%	time between use cases	0.40	3.89%
Transport time	4.28	11.28%	operator exposure time	1.82	17.94%
Distance between seats	5.06	13.32%	number of stops	0.51	5.05%
Number of stops	1.03	2.70%	air circulation	0.80	7.91%
Air circulation	2.08	5.47%	type of loading operation	0.20	1.94%
total:	38.00	100.00%	securing the cargo	0.29	2.80%
			document flow	0.39	3.88%
			type of delivery point	0.46	4.52%
			total:	10.17	100.00%

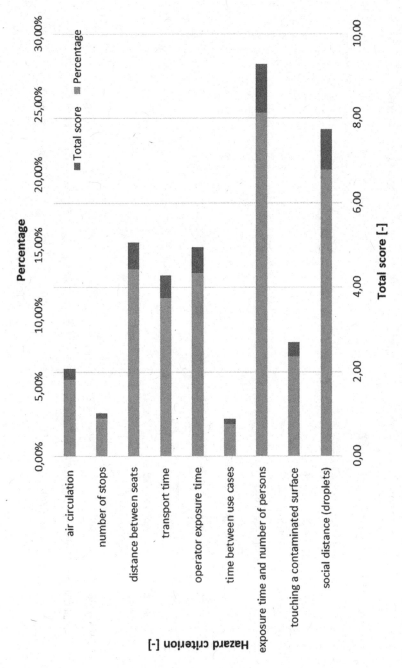

Figure 3.8 Percentage share of the sources of epidemic hazard in passenger transport.

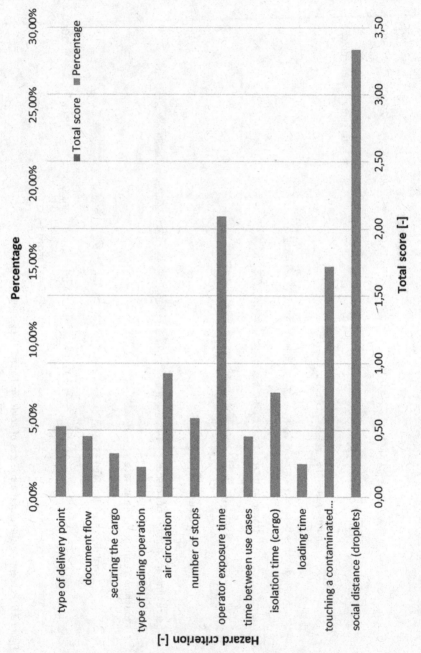

Figure 3.9 Percentage share of the sources of epidemic hazard in freight transport.

The DHI methodology developed by the author is universal in nature, but the results obtained by its application should be adjusted to account for the current infection rate, the rate of tests performed in the given country, or even a region, and the current recommendations for and restrictions imposed on transport, the principles of social distancing and sanitary conditions of work organisation. For this purpose, the following equation has been proposed:

$$h'_{ti} = h_{ti} \cdot m_r \cdot t_p \cdot r_i \cdot d_s \cdot s_c \qquad (3.16)$$

where:

h_{ti} – DHI index (hazard assessment weighted value),
m_r – morbidity rate,
t_p – index of tests performed in a given country or region,
r_i – index of current recommendations and restrictions related to transport,
d_s – index of social distance,
s_c – index of sanitary conditions of work organisation.

3.8 CONCLUSIONS

The methodology developed for the assessment of the epidemic hazard of viral infection using the example of the SARS-CoV-2 coronavirus pandemic, referred to as DHI, enables a detailed analysis of the imminent threats on the basis of process maps and dedicated quantitative scales used to assess the criteria which affect the mechanisms of virus transmission.

The DHI index enables a quantitative multi-criteria weighted assessment of epidemic hazards. In accordance with this methodology, one can scale the range of DHI index values according to the criteria assumed for assessing specific groups of transport services, which affects the possibility of changing the sensitivity and accuracy of the final evaluation.

The DHI index is universal but can also be adjusted to match the current infection rate and related factors.

This approach will enable the DHI index to be adapted to the current general epidemic threat and the preventive actions undertaken. Due to the foregoing, it is possible to conduct periodic analyses which may provide grounds for the development of a forecasting model. Additionally, this will enable regional differentiation of the DHI index on account of the geographical distribution of epidemics that are not global pandemics.

The matrix of hazard assessment for transport services, developed against the threats of the SARS-CoV-2 pandemic, allows for a collective table of hazard factors to be created for a selected group of transport services, consequently making it possible to identify the dominant sources of hazard and to compare services in the context of the risk attributable to epidemic threats. This may constitute the basis for making decisions regarding the selection of transport services or indicate a hierarchy of goals for minimising or eliminating hazard factors, which is the first step in risk management.

The methodology discussed in this monograph will be extended in order to develop a comprehensive methodology dedicated to epidemic risk assessment in transport. For this purpose, studies and analyses are being conducted to estimate the probability of pathogen transmission for specific chains of virus transmission mechanisms via the droplet and contact surface routes. Another field of research pertains to estimation of the effects of the relevant threats as well as the exposure and number of persons potentially at risk. Upon completion of these studies and analyses, a comprehensive risk assessment method will be presented.

Chapter 4

Methodology for Estimating the Probability of Viral Pathogen Transmission in Transport

4.1 GENERAL INFORMATION ON EPIDEMIC MODELS AND THE LIKELIHOOD OF SARS-COV-2 INFECTION

Analysis of the likelihood of viral infections is the very foundation of epidemic modelling. With regard to the SARS-CoV-2 virus pandemic, this often entails modelling of the epidemic progressing at different rates (scenarios). Bearing in mind the functioning of the society during a pandemic, it seems reasonable to isolate healthcare-associated infections, including infections of patients at hospitals and of the medical staff, on account of the different possibilities of reducing contacts in this sector. Other sources of infection are combined into one group. Therefore, the author decided to develop a methodology which would make it possible to isolate an additional group of infections in the transport sector, both in general and in a breakdown into specific groups of transport services.

The most widespread epidemic model is Susceptible-Infected-Recovered (SIR), which represents a system of relationships between S – susceptible individuals, I – infected and infectious individuals, and R – recovered individuals. Unfortunately, one of the assumptions of this and other models is that the incubation period is short enough to disregard it, meaning that a susceptible individual who has become infected falls ill immediately. In the case of the SARS-CoV-2 virus, the incubation period is much longer, and additionally many carriers are asymptomatic. This makes it necessary to apply different epidemic models.

In the study by Shi Chen et al. (2020), an alternative patch dynamic modelling framework has been presented from the perspective of pathogens. Each patch, being the basic module of this modelling framework, includes four standard mechanisms of the pathogen population size change: birth (replication), death, inflow and outflow. This framework naturally distinguishes between-host transmission processes (inflow and outflow) and within-host infection processes (replication) during the entire transmission-infection

DOI: 10.1201/9781003204732-4

cycle. These four mechanisms are sufficiently captured by the discrete time single population patch dynamics model represented by the equation below:

$$P_{i(t+\Delta t)} = P_{it} + \Sigma P_{ji\_inflow} - \Sigma P_{ji\_outflow} + P_{ibirth} + P_{ideath} \qquad (4.1)$$

An interesting probabilistic formalism based on individual-level models (ILMs) that offers rigorous formulas for the probability of infection of individuals, which can be parameterised via maximum likelihood estimation (MLE) applied on compartmental models defined at the population level, has been described by Colubri et al. (2020). The probability of susceptible individual i being infected at time t is expressed as follows (Mahsin et al., 2020):

$$P(i,k,t) = 1 - \exp[(-\Omega_s(i,k) \sum_{j \in C(i,t)} \Omega_T(j,k)\kappa(i,j,t)) - \epsilon(i,k,t)] \qquad (4.2)$$

In this expression, the set of infectious individuals who have interacted with susceptible i in time interval $[t, t + 1]$ is denoted as $C_{(i, t)}$. The risk factors of susceptible individual i becoming infected and infected individual j transmitting the disease are represented by functions $\Omega_S(i)$ and $\Omega_T(j)$, respectively. The time-dependent infection kernel, $\kappa(i,j,t)$, incorporates pairwise risk factors, such as the occurrence and duration of contacts between i and j. The term $\epsilon(i,t)$ can be used to represent other sources of infection. Additionally, one counts the k number of transmission events between susceptible i and infected j, which follows the Poisson distribution with the rate of transmission.

One of the most important parameters used in modelling (predicting) of the spread of an epidemic is reproduction rate R_t, which models the average number of secondary infections at the given time, and which is strongly correlated with current restrictions. A sample model representing the impact of restrictions on the spread of an epidemic has been provided in Flaxman et al. (2020), where the effects of individual restrictions are estimated on the basis of data acquired from many countries. Flaxman et al. (2020) have discussed six interventions, one of which comprises the other five interventions; these are the following:

- timing of school and university closures,
- self-isolating if ill,
- banning of public events,
- any government intervention in place,
- implementing a partial or complete lockdown,
- encouraging social distancing and isolation.

The effect of each intervention is assumed to be multiplicative. $R_{t,m}$ is therefore a function of intervention indicators $I_{k,t,m}$ in place at time t in country m (Flaxman et al., 2020):

$$R_{t,m} = R_{0,m} \cdot e^{-\sum_{k=1}^{6} \alpha_k I_{k,t,m} - \beta_m I_{5,t,m}}$$ (4.3)

where:

$R_{0,m}$ – component of the exponential form to ensure positivity of the reproduction number (it appears outside the exponential),

$I_{k,t,m}$ –indicator variable for intervention k,

α_k – impact of the kth intervention,

β_k – random effect of the kth intervention.

The model proposed by Gogolewski et al. (2020) additionally (besides the death rate data) uses data on testing and new diagnoses, thus ensuring better matching.

Another important parameter is the ratio of people diagnosed daily and the daily number of all infected persons. According to the models provided in Gogolewski et al. (2020), these values demonstrate a median of 0.18 in Poland, which may imply that there are 5.6 undiagnosed and infected persons per every person diagnosed in Poland. This value has a direct effect on the estimation of the infection fatality rate (IFR), which is the probability of death given infection. In many models, the IFR is calculated as a constant for each country. However, where the IFR changes during an epidemic due to reasons such as spread of the disease at different rates among social groups with different IFR, health care quality and change in the quality of treatment over time, milder course of the disease in the late spring season, this may cause the estimation of other parameters to change.

The IFR is derived from the estimates presented in Verity et al. (2020), which assume homogeneous attack rates across age groups. In the paper by Flaxman et al., (2020), in order to better match the estimates of attack rates by age, generated using more detailed information on country and age-specific mixing patterns, the authors have scaled these estimates in the following way. Let c_a be the number of infections generated in age group a, let N_a be the underlying size of the population in that age group and let $AR_a = c_a/N_a$ be the age group-specific attack rate. The adjusted IFR_a is then given by:

$$IFR_a = \frac{AR_{25-44}}{AR_a} \cdot IFR_a'$$ (4.4)

where: AR_{25-44} is the predicted attack rate in the 25–44 years age group.

Verity et al. (2020) and Walker et al. (2020) present calculations performed to obtain overall *IFR* estimates for different age groups in China and countries across Europe, adjusted for both demography and age-specific attack rates.

The model developed by Gogolewski et al. (2020) takes the effects of four types of interventions into account. It was additionally modified to include daily data on the diagnosed cases and extended with the data specific to Poland. Thus developed, the SEIR model assumes that there are four groups in the population:

- *S*: group of people susceptible to infection,
- *E*: group of people exposed to infection, but not infectious,
- *I*: group of people infectious to others in the population,
- *R*: group of people who have ceased to infect, for example, by isolation or recovery. Additionally, recoveries and fatalities across the population are estimated on the basis of the size of the R group.

Consequently, $N=S+E+I+R$, and corresponds to the total population. The basic hypothesis underlying the SEIR model is that all the individuals in the model will perform the four roles as time passes. This model has been used for COVID-19 (S. He et al., 2020; Y.-C. Chen et al., 2020; Tang et al., 2020). S. He et al. (2020) modified the stochastic SEIR model to match COVID-19. The descriptions of the system variables and parameters are provided in Table 4.1, while the relationship between different variables is shown in Figure 4.1.

The modified SEIR model takes two main channels into account. The first one goes to $S - E - I_1 - R$, and the second channel goes to $S - Q - I_2 - H - R$. The first case shows the natural process of the epidemic, and it is a typical SEIR model. The second channel comprises governmental measures of control, including quarantine and hospitalisation. The model presented in S. He et al. (2020) represents nonlinear dynamics of the model.

The $\beta(t)$ transmission rate can be estimated from sample averages calculated over individuals. With reference to the ILM formalism from the previous section, one can note the probability of infection of susceptible i via contact with infected j as follows (Colubri et al., 2020):

$$p_{i,j} = 1 - \exp\left(-\left[a_0 + a_1 X_i\right]\left[b_0 + b_1 Y_j\right]\right) \qquad (4.5)$$

Another example of adaptation of the SEIR model is the application of the Bayesian network (Gogolewski et al., 2020). In this version, the model is based on an assumption that there are five groups in the population, where group *I* is broken down into:

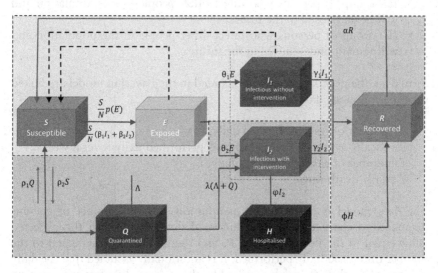

Figure 4.1 Flowchart of the SEIR model proposed in, based on S. He et al. (2020) for COVID-19.

Table 4.1 Descriptions of the SEIR model variables and parameters (based on S. He et al. 2020)

Variable	Description	Parameter	Description
S	Susceptible	α	Temporary immunity rate
E	Exposed	β	Contact and infection rate of transmission per contact from infected class
I_1	Infectious without intervention	p	Probability of transmission per contact from exposed individuals
I_2	Infectious with intervention	θ	Transition rate of exposed individuals to the infected class
R	Recovered	γ	Recovery rate of symptomatic infected individuals to recovered
Q	Quarantined	φ	Rate of the infectious with symptoms to hospitalised
H	Hospitalised	ϕ	Recovered rate of quarantined infected individuals
		λ	Rate of the quarantined class to the recovered class
		ρ	Transition rate of quarantined exposed between the quarantined infected class and the wider community
		Λ	External input from foreign countries

- *ID:* group of persons who infect other people in the population and will be diagnosed in the future,
- *IU:* group of persons who infect other people in the population and will remain undiagnosed in the future.

Moreover, the population groups included in the Bayesian model are linked with the following data:

T: number of tests performed daily,
T_s: locally averaged number of tests performed daily (over a week),
P: number of cases diagnosed daily,
Z: daily death rates.

The data model is based on an assumption that the number of persons diagnosed is characterised by a binomial distribution with the expected value equal to the flow from *I* to *R,* and the number of tests equal to the number of tests actually performed. It is additionally assumed that the daily number of deaths (Z) is characterised by the Poisson distribution.

One of the important parameters of the SEIR model and of its implementations is the frequency with which a susceptible person becomes infected. This parameter links two factors: the probability of being infected upon direct contact with an infected person and the average number of contacts of a susceptible person per a unit of time. On account of the specificity of the SARS-CoV-2 virus and the subject matter of this monograph, which is the risk of viral pathogen transmission in transport, an additional relevant factor determining the frequency of infection is also touching a contaminated surface, which entails virus transmission to the area surrounding the face.

Another approach which assumes that the Gaussian process regression methodology is applied to forecasting as well as to the COVID-19 infections, which may be used in dynamic and chaotic systems, has been presented in Arias Velásquez and Mejía Lara (2020a) and Arias Velásquez and Mejía Lara (2020b).

It is evident that there are many interpretations of the epidemic models, yet all of them share the component of the probabilistic approach. Therefore, the author of this monograph has decided to propose a simplified method for estimating the probability of viral pathogen transmission when using transport services, however, by taking a combination of potential virus transmission mechanisms into account.

4.2 IDENTIFICATION OF THE MECHANISMS OF POTENTIAL VIRAL PATHOGEN TRANSMISSION IN TRANSPORT SERVICES INCLUDING DROPLET AND CONTACT TRANSMISSION

SARS-CoV-2 is perceived to be primarily transmitted via person-to-person contact, through droplets produced while talking, coughing and sneezing. The transmission may also involve other routes, including contaminated surfaces. It is currently accepted that SARS-CoV-2 can be transmitted directly through respiratory droplets or indirectly through fomites (Ong et al., 2020).

The biological details of transmission of beta-coronaviruses (SARS-CoV-2) are known in general terms. These viruses can pass from one individual to another through (Ferretti et al., 2020):

- exhaled droplets,
- aerosol,
- contamination of surfaces,
- possibly through faecal-oral contamination.

There is still much uncertainty about the SARS-CoV-2 transmission route. According to the New Coronavirus Pneumonia Diagnosis and Treatment Plan published by the Chinese National Health Commission, the main human-to-human transmission routes are close contacts (direct/indirect) and large respiratory droplets produced by coughing or sneezing, or droplets of saliva, but the aerosol and faecal-oral transmission could not be excluded and need further investigation (Zhang et al., 2020).

According to the World Health Organization (2020), considering the current evidence, the COVID-19 virus is transmitted between people through respiratory droplets and contact routes. Droplet transmission occurs when a person is in close contact (within 1 m) with someone who displays respiratory symptoms (e.g. coughing or sneezing), and is therefore at risk of having their mucosae (mouth and nose) or conjunctivae (eyes) exposed to potentially infective respiratory droplets (which are generally considered to be > 5–10 µm in diameter). Droplet transmission may also occur through fomites in the immediate environment around the infected person. Therefore, the COVID-19 virus transmission can occur by direct contact with infected people and by indirect contact with surfaces in the immediate environment or with objects used by/on the infected person.

Airborne transmission is different from droplet transmission as it refers to the presence of microbes within droplet nuclei, which are generally considered to be particles < 5 µm in diameter, and which result from the evaporation of larger droplets or exist within dust particles. They may remain in the air for long periods of time, and can be transmitted to others over distances greater than 1 m. Based on a report of the WHO-China Joint Mission on Coronavirus Disease 2019, comprising an analysis of 75,465 COVID-19 cases in China, no airborne transmission was reported.

Additionally, the probability of viral pathogen transmission depends on factors such as exposure time, distance, ventilation, number of surfaces potentially contaminated by the pathogen and frequency of human contact with these surfaces or skin-to-skin contact. Furthermore, the probability of the pathogen transmission is affected by the personal protective equipment in use, including face masks and gloves, as well as regular cleaning and disinfection of both touch surfaces and hands. Wearing a mask is found to be much more useful than washing hands for control of the influenza A virus in the tested office setting. Regular cleaning of high-touch surfaces, which can reduce the infection risk by 2.14%, is recommended and is much more efficient than hand washing (Zhang and Li, 2018).

In order to reduce the likelihood of droplet transmission, the principle of social distancing is commonly applied. It is currently assumed that the safe distance to be maintained is 1.5–2 m; however, as the relevant data imply, the virus can spread on sneezing over a distance of up to 3.5 m, and on coughing it is up to 6.5 m , as indicated by a computational fluid dynamics model (Ansys Fluent) developed to study the behaviour of droplets containing the virus (Shafaghi et al., 2020b; Xie et al., 2007). The equation used to calculate the horizontal travel distance of the SARS-CoV-2 virus has been provided in Chapter 3 (Equation 3.3).

Nande et al. (2020) have provided a stochastic SEIR epidemic model to examine the effects of the COVID-19 clinical progression and transmission network structure on the outcomes of social distancing interventions.

Consequently, the viral pathogen transmission probability determined on the basis of the ratio of the infected should be considered due to the area congestion. The total area consists of three zones: crowded zone, mild zone and uncrowded zone, with different infection probabilities characterised by the number of people gathered there (Karako et al., 2020). If one is to apply this approach in means of transport, and particularly in collective transport, attention should also be paid to the diverse potential virus transmission routes. Highly crowded means of transport are characterised by a high risk of infection by droplets, contact with a contaminated surface, or direct contact by touch. Consequently, the infection likelihood is by far the highest in this case. When adequate distance between passengers (Mild Zone) is maintained, the mechanism of virus transmission by touch with another person can actually be excluded. What is also reduced by that means is the risk of droplet transmission and the quantity of potentially contaminated surfaces. Therefore, in this case, the probability of infection can be assumed as moderate. With regard to individual transport, the virus transmission by touch contact with another person should be eliminated in advance, and in practical terms, the droplet route can also be excluded, which leaves the possibility of virus transmission through contaminated (by a previous passenger) surfaces, the risk of which is by far the lowest. The virus transmission mechanisms for different levels of congestion in public spaces (including in means of transport) along with an illustration of the levels of viral pathogen transmission probability $(p_{i,j})$ and the consequences in terms of the growth of the infected population are provided in Figure 4.2.

It is possible to increase the distance between passengers in means of collective transport by limiting the number of passengers who can travel by the given vehicle at the same time. This is precisely the solution typically applied under social restrictions with the purpose of limiting the number of passengers using collective public transport to 50% of the number of seats or 30% of the total vehicle capacity.

Besides the distance between passengers, another important factor affecting the probability of the pathogen transmission is contact with an infected person or the duration of exposure to pathogens (including airborne and surface transmission). However, the conclusion arising from analysis of droplet transmission is that the longer one remains in a vicinity of an infected person (including an asymptomatic individual), the higher the

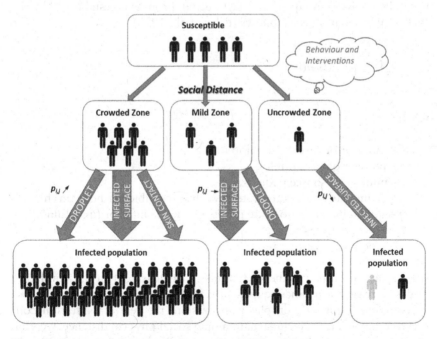

Figure 4.2 Illustration of the mechanisms and probability of viral pathogen transmission in public spaces, including in means of transport.

probability of viral pathogen transmission. According to surveys of travelling by means of public transport, this probability increases on average by 0.15% with every consecutive hour of travel (Hu et al., 2020).

For example, Ko et al. (2004) have estimated the risk of tuberculosis transmission on a typical commercial airliner using a simple one box model and a sequential box model. This implies that the risk and incidence decrease sharply in a stepwise fashion in cabins downstream of the cabin containing the source case, assuming some potential for airflow from more contaminated to less contaminated cabins. This analysis comprises a high efficiency particulate air (HEPA) filter installed on-board the airplane. Schultz and Fuchte (2020) have presented an evaluation of aircraft boarding scenarios considering reduced transmission risks, having implemented a transmission model in a virtual aircraft environment to evaluate individual interactions between passengers during aircraft boarding and deboarding.

Ventilation has been widely recognised as an efficient engineering control measure for airborne transmission (Melikov et al., 2020). A growing number of epidemiological cases provide for the possibility of airborne transmission (not only by droplets) of coronavirus diseases. Dai and Zhao (2020) obtained the quantum generation rate produced by a COVID-19 infector with a reproductive number-based fitting approach, and then estimated the association between infection probability and ventilation rate using the Wells–Riley equation. The infection probability established by the Wells–Riley equation is as follows (Riley et al., 1978):

$$p = \frac{C}{S} = 1 - e^{-Iqpt/Q} \tag{4.6}$$

where:

C – number of cases to develop infection,
S – number of susceptibles,
I – number of source patients,
p – pulmonary ventilation rate of each susceptible per hour (m³/h),
q – quantum generation rate produced by one infector (quantum/h),
t – exposure time (h),
Q – room ventilation rate (m³/h).

If both the infectors and the susceptibles wear masks, then the ventilation rate is increased four times equivalently.

Assuming respiratory-droplet transmission, the relevant infection control recommendations include maintaining social/physical distance, wearing masks, case isolation and contact tracing (Pitol and Julian, 2020). As presented in Dai and Zhao (2020), if people wear masks, natural ventilation or normal mechanical ventilation can provide enough ventilation rate to ensure the infection probability of less than 1%.

Table 4.2 lists the corresponding air change rates. The air change rate is a measure of how much fresh/clean air replaces indoor air within 1 h.

In accordance with the current legislation, people are obliged to wear face masks or cover their mouths and noses in public spaces, and these include means of collective transport. Given the data concerning the virus of influenza, one can conclude how important the wearing of masks is in terms of the spread of viruses. The likelihood of being infected with influenza is 8.75%, but with the obligatory masks, this probability drops to 3.82% (Zhang and Li, 2018). Consequently, the likelihood of influenza infection decreases about 2.55 times assuming that people wear masks. The total risk of influenza transmission can even be reduced from 8.75% to 0.45% if the N95-type mask is worn tightly sealed by the infected person (Zhang and Li, 2018). With regard to the foregoing, one can conclude that wearing masks reduces the likelihood of droplet viral infection. Additionally, wearing masks also contributes to reducing the likelihood of infection by touch. Masks partially block the particles released by a sick person, which could drop on the given surface then to be touched by other users.

Although the risk of the SARS-CoV-2 transmission via fomites is estimated to be low, a person's infection risk increases when accounting for the hundreds of objects with which people are in contact every hour,

Table 4.2 Air change rate requirement for the expected SARS-CoV-2 infection probability and wearing mask in means of transport (Y – with mask, N – without mask) (based on Dai and Zhao 2020)

Infection probability		Bus		Aircraft cabin	
	Volume (m³)	75		100	
	Exposure time (h)	0.5		4	
	Air change rates (/h)				
	quantum generation rate of 14/h	With mask	Without mask	With mask	Without mask
2.0%		0.33	1.3	2	8
1.0%		0.7	2.8	4	16
0.1%		7	27	35	160
2.0%	quantum generation rate of 48/h	1.2	4.8	7	30
1.0%		2.4	9.6	15	55
0.1%		24	93	125	550

and further thousands of frequently contacted objects (buttons in public transport). Each interaction provides an opportunity for SARS-CoV-2 transmission. The risk of infection from multiple contacts with fomites is substantially higher.

The factors considered relevant with regard to infection by contact with a contaminated surface or with an infected person include the material the surface is made of, cleaning and disinfection, as well as frequency of contact with the surface. The more often the given surface is touched, the more likely it is to be infectious. Moreover, viruses remain on surfaces made of different materials for different periods of time. According to the Australian CSIRO agency, the virus persists on touch surfaces such as banknotes, mobile phones and touchscreens for up to 28 days. On plastic surfaces, it can persist for up to 72 h, on steel surfaces – up to 48 h, and on cardboard surfaces – up to 24 h (Patients et al., 2020). What also matters is that in order to become infected by touch, a healthy person would have to touch the contaminated surface and then transfer the virus from the hand to the mucous membranes, for instance, by touching the mouth, nose or eye area.

Viruses can reach the mucous membrane if a person touches the mouth, nasopharynx and eyes with a contaminated hand. Studies have shown that the mean rate of all-finger contacts with the lips, nostrils and eyes ranges from 0.7 h^{-1} to 15 h^{-1}. In the study by Zhang and Li (2018), it was estimated that the virus transfer rate from the fingertip to the mucous membranes is 35% and the quantity of virus ($TCID_{50}$ – Median Tissue Culture Infectious Dose) on all analysed surfaces ceases to increase rapidly after 3 h. The transfer rate between hands and various surfaces directly determines the amount of pathogen transmitted via the fomite route. The dose-response parameter based on intranasal inoculation of humans $\alpha_1 = 5.7 \times 10^{-5}$ $TCID_{50}^{-1}$.

As stated in the study by Zhang and Li (2018), approximately 4.2% of the influenza infection risk comes from fomites. However, for other infectious diseases, such as COVID-19, it can be different. Results of this research show that the long-range airborne, fomite and close contact routes contribute to 54.3%, 4.2% and 44.5% of influenza infections, respectively.

The SARS-CoV-2 virus spreads by hand–mouth pathways or by skin-borne and eye infections, which transfer from hands to skin or eyes from sources including natural flora of the skin, and nasal passages. Figure 4.3 presents this viral pathogen transmission mechanism, and includes dose and transfer efficiency reduction by surface disinfection of the surface. Ryan et al. (2014) focused on transfer efficiencies as well as on surface occurrence data and the percentage transfer of pathogen from skin to skin or hand to mouth/eye. The risk of infection was computed using an exponential dose–response beta-Poisson model:

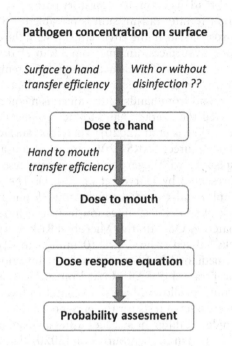

Figure 4.3 Scenario for calculating the exposure and risk associated with fomite contamination. Exposure to microorganisms on fomites was modelled as associated with a single touch of the fomite, followed by transfer to the mouth.

$$r_i = 1 - \left[1 + \frac{d}{N_{50}}\left(2^{\frac{1}{\alpha}} - 1\right)\right]^{-\alpha}$$

(4.7)

where:

d – dose,
N_{50}, α – model parameters.

As mentioned in Pitol and Julian (2020), the authors used the Quantitative Microbial Risk Assessment framework to examine the risks of community transmission of SARS-CoV-2 through contaminated surfaces and to evaluate the effectiveness of hand and surface disinfection as potential interventions. The risks posed by contacting surfaces in communities are low (average of the median risks 1.6×10^{-4} – 5.6×10^{-9}) for the community infection prevalence rates ranging between 0.2% and 5%. Indirect transmission via fomites contributes to the spread of common respiratory pathogens, and the evidence to date suggests that fomite transmission is possible for SARS-CoV-2. The infective coronavirus persists in the environment, with the experimental evidence of persistence on surfaces ranging from 3 h to 28 days, depending on such environmental factors as the surface material and temperature (Riddell et al., 2020). Viruses readily transfer from contaminated surfaces to the hand upon contact, and from hands to the mucous membranes on the face. Studies have reported the average hand-to-face contacts ranging from 16 to 37 times an hour (Lewis et al., 2020). Therefore, surface contamination could pose a risk of indirect SARS-CoV-2 transmission and also needs to be considered, especially with regard to transport processes. An interesting study has been presented by Harvey et al. (2021). The authors collected surface swab samples and recorded touches on 33 unique surfaces at 12 locations. The risk of COVID-19 infection from touching a contaminated surface was estimated by Quantitative Microbial Risk Assessment (QMRA). The infection risks ranged from 2 per 10 million to 4 per 10 thousand (mean=6.5×10^{-5}, median=2.2×10^{-6}). The risk of infection was estimated based on the concentration of SARS-CoV-2 on surfaces, assuming a single hand-to-surface contact followed by a single hand-to-face contact.

Some interesting results of tests for the presence of the SARS-CoV-2 virus performed on samples of different surfaces using an example of a passenger ship have been discussed in Mouchtouri et al. (2020). The authors collected environmental samples from a ferryboat while investigating the ongoing COVID-19 outbreak with an attack rate of 31.3% (119/380 travellers). The air and surface samples were collected according to the World Health Organization guidelines (World Health Organization, 2020). All samples were tested by the real-time reverse transcriptase–polymerase chain reaction (RT-PCR). The SARS-CoV-2 RNA was detected on the air exhaust duct surface and on the screen of the exhaust duct leading from the ship hospital and cabins to the open deck. Respiratory droplets/nuclei from the infected persons were displaced and deposited on the air duct and screen of the ship air exhaust located on the open deck, three decks above the ship hospital's examination area. The air from cabins and toilets of symptomatic and asymptomatic patients were carried to the same air exhaust duct.

4.3 METHODOLOGY FOR ESTIMATING THE TOTAL PROBABILITY OF VIRAL PATHOGEN TRANSMISSION IN TRANSPORT SERVICES

Having analysed different epidemic models, one can conclude that, regardless of the adopted approach, each of them is based on estimating and forecasting the probability of virus transmission. An important parameter determining their correlations with the reality is the size of the susceptible and the infected sets. In order to estimate the quantitative values of these sets as precisely as possible, one should primarily analyse all possible mechanisms of virus transmission from a person to another. There are individual studies elaborating on the subject of the probability of viral infection in transport, described earlier in the monograph, but they concern selected means of transport and are almost entirely limited to passenger transport. Furthermore, this probability is often calculated on the basis of models of pathogen spread in a confined space of the means of transport, represented by advanced mathematical functions. The aforementioned conditions make it difficult to adapt the said models to other means of transport, or even virtually impossible to translate them into other types of transport services, excluding transport of goods. This is precisely why the author of this monograph decided to develop a universal methodology for estimating the probability of viral pathogen transmission by referring to the SARS-CoV-2 pandemic, assuming full mathematical disclosure and an open process formula, aimed to make it possible to take specific other mechanisms of virus transmission into account when providing transport services.

Böhmer et al. (2020) investigated the COVID-19 outbreak in Germany resulting from a single travel-associated primary case. Case interviews were performed to describe the timing of the onset and the nature of symptoms, and to identify and classify contacts as high risk (one had cumulative face-to-face contact with a confirmed case for ≥15 min, direct contact with secretions or body fluids of a patient with confirmed COVID-19). The relevant finding was that the overall secondary attack rate was below 10% for close contacts. Even prolonged meeting situations left some people without a transmission, while on another occasion a transmission happened when a pre-symptomatic person sat back to back with another person and handed over a salt dispenser. This demonstrates the relevance of even short contacts with contagious people. An Italian study on the outbreak of COVID-19 (Lavezzo et al., 2020) showed that the number of asymptomatic cases was roughly 45% out of the entire number of cases. This means that even if symptomatic passengers are removed from travel, the probability of having contagious passengers should still be considered if the virus is active in the population and pre-symptomatic passengers are contagious. In the study presented by X. He et al. (2020), the incubation period was estimated at 5.2 days on average, and the onset of infectiousness was estimated at 2 days before the occurrence of symptoms. A higher probability of infection is estimated at ca. 12 h before the onset of symptoms. Another important factor is the time for which the virus can survive on different fomites (contact surfaces in means of transport or loads). Therefore, the contagiousness of surfaces touched by multiple passengers is a matter of concern. It should be mentioned that the overall contribution of contact transmission to the total transmission is currently deemed low.

Consequently, the key factors of the epidemic spread were analysed to evaluate the contribution of different transmission routes.

For purposes of the methodology proposed for the determination of the likelihood of viral pathogen transmission in transport services against the context of passenger or customer exposure in freight transport, the potential mechanisms of pathogen transmission for activities performed consecutively while providing the given service were identified. Three possible virus transmission mechanisms have been taken into account:

- droplet transmission,
- surface contact,
- direct contact with another person.

For each transport service, adequate assumptions were adopted with regard to travelling time, distance, contact surfaces and applicable regulations. Next, based on an analysis of the chain of events resulting from the process mapping (Chapter 3), all activities including the potential virus transmission mechanisms were identified. The outcome of this procedure was a set of independent events to which, with reference to the literature review, it is possible to assign the values of probability of elementary events. The final stage was estimating the total probability of viral pathogen transmission for the given transport service (Figure 4.4).

The assumption underlying the method developed by the author is that it can be adapted to specific conditions of individual transport services, making it possible to establish the values of probability for these services instead of averaging them for the entire transport sector or breaking it down into passenger and freight transport. This allows for a comparative analysis of individual types of transport services and for considering other events taking place during the performance of the transport process which may be sources of virus transmission. Therefore, different potential situations were considered for individual transport services, such as paying or buying a ticket, taking a seat or a standing place, holding luggage, touching the cargo or surfaces in means of transport (e.g. seats, railings and handles). Also the potential distances between those participating in the transport process were analysed and distinguished, taking the specifics of the given service into account, as they affect the mechanisms of virus transmission, either via droplets or by direct contact (touch). Another parameter taken into consideration when establishing the probability of elementary events occurring in transport services, assuming average values of time for specific activities conducted in respective processes, representative of the given transport service, is exposure time.

All of the foregoing makes the probability values determined by that means strongly oriented towards the specificity of individual transport services, corresponding to real random events which may lead to viral pathogen transmission in transport.

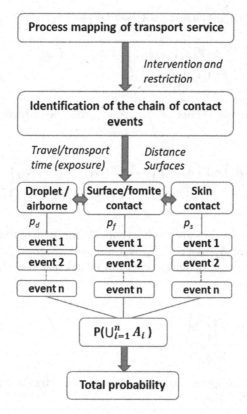

Figure 4.4 Algorithm of the methodology for determination of the total probability of viral pathogen transmission in transport processes.

In order to calculate the total probability of viral pathogen transmission in the given transport service, the author used the definition of probability of a sum of independent events.

A sum of events is understood as a random event which takes place when at least one of its constituent events takes place. The sum n of consecutive events A_i, where $i = 1,...,n$, can be expressed as follows: $\bigcup_{i=1}^{n} A_i$ or $A_1 u A_2 u A_3 u ... u A_n$.

The probability of the n sum of events is expressed by what is referred to as the inclusion–exclusion formula, which assumes the following form:

$$P\left(\bigcup_{i=1}^{n} A_i\right) = P\left(A_1 \cup A_2 \cup A_3 \cup \ldots \cup A_n\right) = P\left(A_1\right) + P\left(A_2\right) + \ldots$$
$$+ P\left(A_n\right) - P\left(A_1 \cap A_2\right) - \ldots + P\left(A_1 \cap A_2 \cap A_3\right)$$
$$+ \ldots - P\left(A_1 \cap A_2 \cap A_3 \cap A_4\right) - \ldots \tag{4.8}$$

For example, for the events of A_1, A_2, A_3, the above formula is noted as follows:

$$P\left(A_1 \cup A_2 \cup A_3\right) = P\left(A_1\right) + P\left(A_2\right) + P\left(A_3\right) - P\left(A_1 \cap A_2\right)$$
$$- P\left(A_1 \cap A_3\right) - P\left(A_2 \cap A_3\right) + P\left(A_1 \cap A_2 \cap A_3\right)$$

The independent events are such events A_i for which their intersection, i.e. the product of $A_1 \cap A_2 \cap \ldots \cap A_n$, is a null set. Where this is the case, the probability of the sum of such events can be calculated using the following formula:

$$P\left(\bigcup_{i=1}^{n} A_i\right) = 1 - P\left(\bigcap_{i=1}^{n} A_i'\right) \tag{4.9}$$

The A_i' events are opposite to events A_i, which is why their probability can be expressed as follows:

$$P\left(A_i'\right) = 1 - P(A_i) \tag{4.10}$$

Since events A_i are independent, it implies that the opposite A_i' events are also independent, and hence the probability of the product of independent events A_i' in formula 4.9.

The probability of the product of independent events is expressed by the following formula:

$$P\left(\bigcap_{i=1}^{n} A_i'\right) = \prod_{i=1}^{n} P\left(A_i'\right) = P\left(A_1'\right) * P\left(A_2'\right) * \ldots * P\left(A_n'\right) \tag{4.11}$$

Therefore, by combining equations 4.10 and 4.11, one obtains the following formula for calculating the probability of the sum of n independent events:

$$P\left(\bigcup_{i=1}^{n} A_i\right) = 1 - \prod_{i=1}^{n}\left(1 - P\left(A_i\right)\right) \qquad (4.12)$$

The above formula can also be transformed into the following form:

$$P\left(\bigcup_{i=1}^{n} A_i\right) = 1 - \left(1 - P\left(A_1\right)\right)\left(1 - P\left(A_2\right)\right)...\left(1 - P\left(A_n\right)\right) \qquad (4.13)$$

The probability of being infected with the virus is also affected by the number of infected persons in the population. This value also determine the volume of viral pathogens around us. For example, according to the data provided by the Ministry of Health on 30 November 2020, there had been 990,811 diagnosed cases of infection in Poland since the onset of the pandemic. This number corresponds to ca. 2.6% of Poland's population. The number of active diagnosed cases was 396,147 on that day, which represented ca. 1.04% of the population. However, one should also consider the fact that there are undiagnosed cases in the population. Scientists from the Faculty of Mathematics, Informatics and Mechanics of the University of Warsaw (Gogolewski et al., 2020) established the ratio of daily undiagnosed cases to those diagnosed at 5.6. This implies that the actual total number of infected persons may be more than five times that of the confirmed number of cases. Additionally, according to a model which considers the entire year of the pandemic and accounts for its seasonal nature, developed by the University of Warsaw, the number of cases diagnosed in Poland by 17 March 2021 will have come to 3,928,701, which corresponds to 10.24% of the total Polish population (Gogolewski et al., 2020).

Given the current pandemic situation, being the actual motivation for elaborating upon the subject matter addressed in this monograph and, at the same time, representing the case study used to verify the method proposed, the research also took some general recommendations and the social behaviour patterns into consideration in light of the SARS-CoV-2 pandemic. However, it should be noted that if the methodology developed by the author is to be applied to other epidemics, the current legal status and social behaviour patterns must be updated. Since the regulations in force require people to cover their mouths and noses in public spaces, it has been assumed that all those participating in the transport services described below indeed wear masks on their faces. Nevertheless, the analysis of the transport services in question comprises viral pathogen transmission probabilities for the cases of the masks being and not being worn. Using data on the functioning of face masks vis-à-vis the transmission of the influenza virus, the probability of droplet infection was reduced 2.55 times (Zhang and Li, 2018).

Indirect transmission via fomites (contaminated surfaces) contributes to the spread of common respiratory pathogens (Boone and Gerba, 2007), and the evidence to date suggests that fomite transmission is possible for SARS-CoV-2. The surface-to-hand transfer and the hand-to-mucous membrane transfer were both assumed proportional to the virus concentration on the contaminated surface and its transfer efficiency at both interfaces. In order to estimate the probability of virus transmission by touch, the author assumed the values reported in the studies by Pitol and Julian (2020) to determine distributions of the probability of infection by touching contaminated surfaces depending on the touching frequency as well as the prevalence in the given population.

Following an analysis of the literature data and the results of the research completed to date (Pitol and Julian, 2020) for the elementary events in which a random event of the virus transmission by touching a contaminated surface may occur, a table was compiled with the values of infection probability dependent on the share of infected individuals in the population (prevalence rate). Moreover, analogically to the instance of wearing masks in the analysis of droplet virus transmission, the probability values were provided for hand disinfection (assuming the metric of 50% of the population) or surface disinfection by the transport operator (twice a day) (Table 4.3).

The infection probability of 10^{-6} is equivalent to one person infected as a consequence of hand-to-mouth contact per every million persons touching the surface. The overwhelming majority of interactions with fomites is

Table 4.3 Average median probability of infection from fomite contact for different prevalence rates and disinfection scenarios (based on Pitol and Julian (2020)

Frequency of contact with surface	No hand or surface disinfection	Hand disinfection	Surface disinfection
0.2% prevalence rate			
High contact frequency (at least three times per hour)	10^{-8}	10^{-10}	10^{-14}
Low contact frequency (not more than once per 1–4 h]	10^{-8}	10^{-11}	10^{-23}
1.0% prevalence rate			
High contact frequency (at least three times per hour)	10^{-6}	10^{-9}	10^{-7}
Low contact frequency (not more than once per 1–4 h)	10^{-7}	10^{-9}	10^{v10}
5.0% prevalence rate			
High contact frequency (at least three times per hour)	10^{-4}	10^{-7}	10^{-4}
Low contact frequency (not more than once per 1–4 h)	10^{-5}	10^{-7}	10^{-8}

associated with probability $< 10^{-4}$ (equivalent to one person infected per ten thousand people touching the surface). That is why, in most analyses of the transport-related infection risk, the probability of virus transmission by touching the surface is completely ignored. And yet the author of this monograph had decided to include it in the methodology proposed on account of various reasons, including the risk estimation vis-à-vis the daily country-wide hazard rates, where the number of people exposed to infection was considerably higher.

The analysis of transport processes made it possible to establish the frequency of contact with different surfaces depending on the transport service type.

Similarly to all respiratory infectious diseases, the present COVID-19 pandemic is a warning that close contact should be avoided on account of the droplet and airborne virus transmission routes activated in respiratory activities.

When estimating the probability of viral infection via droplets, social distance and time of exposure to the pathogen are considered very important parameters. For transport services, this should relate to the distance between passengers or customers in freight transport and the time of travel or of contact between the participants in the freight transport process. On account of the generally accepted assumption that the main mechanism of the SARS-CoV-2 virus transmission involves droplets, many studies published to date have addressed the impact of distance and exposure time. A popular approach comprises models based on the Wells–Riley model used to quantify the effects of social distancing on the risk of infection. The Wells–Riley model is one of the most classical and popular models allowing for the infection risk to be predicted. The method developed by the author adapts the distributions of probability established with reference to the results of the research by Sun and Zhai (2020). They analysed the statistics and distributions of droplets with different sizes and in various numbers during a standard conversation using experimental field data and considering the air distribution effectiveness given a specific ventilation factor. The model thus developed was calibrated and verified by considering the results obtained for bus passengers forming a representative case in terms of the initial infection rate (2.17 %), the duration of stay and the number of occupants. Infective quantum q in the modified model was subsequently calibrated with reference to this case. The distance between two passengers on-board the bus was estimated at 1.05 m, and the actual occupancy rate was ca. 42%.

Based on the above studies, tables of the infection probability were prepared, and specific functions of droplet infection probability were assumed, conditional on the exposure time for selected means of transport and interior rooms, considering 100% and 50% occupancy of the available places (Tables 4.4 and 4.5 and Figures 4.5 and 4.6).

Table 4.4 Probability of infection in means of transport for different exposure times and passenger occupancy rates (based on Sun and Zhai 2020)

Means of transport	*Exposure time*							
	5 [min]	10 [min]	15 [min]	20 [min]	25 [min]	30 [min]	500 [min]	1,000 [min]
Train (100% occu.)	0.0117	0.0233	0.0350	0.0467	0.0583	0.0700	0.7000	0.9000
Train (50% occu.)	0.0083	0.0167	0.0250	0.0333	0.0417	0.0500	0.6200	0.8200
Public bus (100% occu.)	0.0300	0.0600	0.0900	0.1200	0.1500	0.1800	0.9800	1.0000
Public bus (50% occu.)	0.0225	0.0450	0.0675	0.0900	0.1125	0.1350	0.9500	1.0000
Airplane (100% occu.)	0.0102	0.0203	0.0305	0.0407	0.0508	0.0610	0.6000	0.9000
Airplane (50% occu.)	0.0082	0.0163	0.0245	0.0327	0.0408	0.0490	0.5400	0.8000
Underground railway (100% occu.)	0.0200	0.0400	0.0600	0.0800	0.1000	0.1200	0.8500	0.9800
Underground railway (50% occu.)	0.0125	0.0250	0.0375	0.0500	0.0625	0.0750	0.7400	0.9500
Regular coach service (100% occu.)	0.0124	0.0248	0.0372	0.0496	0.0620	0.0744	0.7400	0.9500
Regular coach service (50% occu.)	0.0101	0.0202	0.0303	0.0404	0.0505	0.0606	0.6000	0.8500

And again, based on the relevant process maps and the identified chains of elementary (contact) events, individual activities involving a possibility of a random event with a potential mechanism of droplet virus transmission as well as their average duration times were determined. Next, in the above tables and figures, the values of infection probability were read each time for the pre-assumed travel time or contact activity in freight transport for the given means of transport (or room), and then they were assigned the corresponding values of probability of elementary events.

The final measure of the likelihood of viral pathogen transmission was the probability of a sum of all independent elementary events identified in the process.

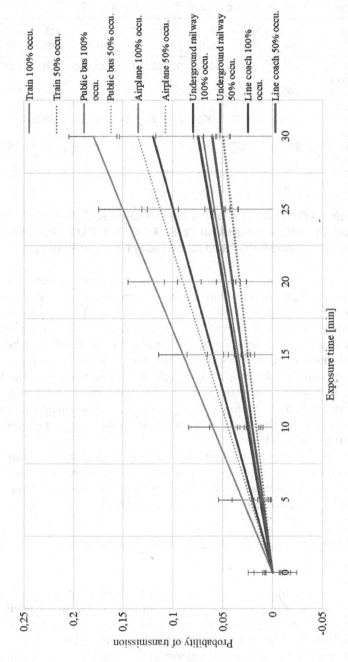

Figure 4.5 Probability of viral pathogen transmission in means of transport for exposure times ranging at 0–30 min and different passenger occupancy rates.

Table 4.5 Probability of infection in public spaces (rooms) for different exposure times and people occupancy rates (based on Sun and Zhai, 2020)

Exposure time Rooms	5 [min]	10 [min]	15 [min]	20 [min]	25 [min]	30 [min]	500 [min]	1,000 [min]
Office (small) (100% occu.)	0.0042	0.0083	0.0125	0.0167	0,0208	0.0250	0.3000	0.5500
Office (small) (50% occu.)	0,0028	0.0056	0.0084	0.0111	0.0139	0.0167	0.1800	0.3500
Classroom (100% occu.)	0.0167	0.0333	0.0500	0.0667	0.0833	0.1000	0.8800	0.9800
Classroom (50% occu.)	0.0128	0.0257	0.0385	0.0513	0.0642	0.0770	0.7800	0.9200

4.4 COMPILATION AND COMPARISON OF VIRAL PATHOGEN TRANSMISSION PROBABILITIES FOR VARIOUS TRANSPORT SERVICES (PASSENGER AND FREIGHT TRANSPORT)

In order to calculate the total probability of viral pathogen transmission in specific groups of transport services, a map of the service delivery process should be drawn up in the first step, considering all the activities which involve pathogen transmission mechanisms (Chapter 3). Then, applying the aforementioned methodology, one could calculate the probability of the sum of all independent elementary events identified in the process, involving viral pathogen transmission by droplets or touch. According to the methodology proposed, one should also take into account the factors and parameters affecting pathogen transmission, such as distance, disinfection and exposure time, considering whether those who participate in the transport process are wearing protective masks.

In order to demonstrate the procedure followed while implementing the methodology in question, a detailed case study has been provided, similarly to the previous chapter, addressing three types of transport services: collective public transport, car sharing and courier services.

4.4.1 Case Study of Collective Public Transport

4.4.1.1 General Assumptions

According to current restrictions, wearing masks or covering the mouth and nose is mandatory. Consequently, one should assume that passengers, drivers and other participants in the transport service wear masks on their faces. Additionally, the bus or tram driver remains in an isolated zone, separated from the passenger compartment by a glass panel or another

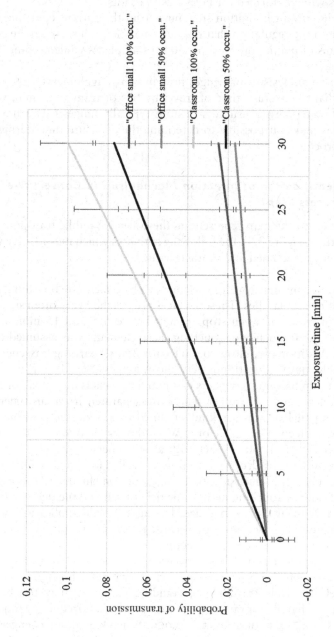

Figure 4.6 Probability of viral pathogen transmission in public spaces (rooms) for exposure times ranging at 0–30 min and different people occupancy rates.

shield. In order to demonstrate the differences in the viral pathogen transmission probability values in cases with masks being or not being worn, calculations were performed for both these variants.

Another important limitation stemming from the current epidemic situation is due to the regulation that only up to 50% of all seats can be occupied in means of public transport, or 30% of all places while keeping 50% of seats free.

Based on an analysis of passenger flow in urban agglomerations, it was estimated that the average time of travel by bus or tram is 25 min, while the time of travel between successive stops typically ranges between 5 and 15 min. This makes it possible to determine the exposure time during the transport process.

4.4.1.2 Identification of Infection Mechanisms in Consecutive Process Steps

With reference to the map representing the collective public transport process (Chapter 3, Figure 3.3), the following activities which may involve virus transmission were defined and characterised:

1 Boarding: one may touch the elements which facilitate boarding, such as railings or handles. These surfaces are touched very often since the time of travel between stops ranges between 5 and 15 min, which is why the frequency of touching these elements was assumed to be high. Additionally, close contact with other boarding passengers is possible, but its duration is very short, i.e. less than 1 min.
2 Ticket purchasing: passengers can purchase tickets at a kiosk or from a ticket machine. Since the sellers are separated from customers by a glass panel or another kind of shield in kiosks, the possibility of droplet infection is ruled out. When buying a ticket at the ticket machine, there is no contact with another person, which eliminates the possibility of droplet infection as well. However, in both cases one can become infected by touching a contaminated surface, or more specifically by touching money, the ticket itself and the ticket machine screen. A ticket can be purchased using a mobile application, which eliminates the risk of infection because it does not require contact with another person or any infrastructure.
3 Validating the ticket: when validating a ticket, it is not necessary to touch the vehicle elements or contact other people directly.
4 Travelling: while travelling, a standing passenger may touch such objects as handles or railings, i.e., surfaces that are frequently touched, and is also at risk of droplet infection. When seated, a passenger typically does not touch any parts of the vehicle with hands.

5 Deboarding: one may touch certain elements of the vehicle such as handles or railings, which are frequently touched surfaces. Contemporarily, the vehicle doors are opened at stops by drivers, which is why passengers do not have to press any button to do so. Close contact with other deboarding passengers is possible, but its time is very short – less than 1 min.

4.4.1.3 Analysis of the Process Scenarios (Variants)

4.4.1.3.1 Variant 1

The passenger takes a standing place having purchased the ticket at the kiosk before boarding the vehicle (Table 4.6).

Next, following the adopted computational procedure (formulae 4.8–4.13), the following values are calculated, one by one:

$$P(A_2 \text{ u } A_3) = 1 - 0{,}999*0.9900 = 0.010099$$

$$P(A_5 \text{ u } A_6) = 1 - 0.999*0.8875 = 0.1126$$

$$P(A_7 \text{ u } A_8) = 1 - 0.999*0.9900 = 0.010099$$

Finally, having made the relevant substitutions in formula 4.13, one could obtain the total probability for the variant in which passengers do not wear protective masks:

$$P = 1 - (1\text{-}0.0001){\cdot}(1\text{-}0.010099){\cdot}(1\text{-}0.1126){\cdot}(1\text{-}0.010099)$$
$$= 0.1305 = 13.05\%$$

Next, following the computational procedure (formulae 4.8–4.13), the following values are calculated (Table 4.7), one by one:

Table 4.6 Probabilities of elementary events occurring in means of collective public transport – variant 1: without masks

Event	Transmission route	P(Ai)	1-P(Ai)	P	1-P
Ticket purchase	Contact	0.0001	0.9999	0.0001	0.9999
Boarding	Contact	0.0001	0.9999	0.0101	0.9899
	Droplet	0.0100	0.9900		
Ticket validation	-----	-----	-----	-----	-----
Travelling	Contact	0.0001	0.9999	0.1126	0.8874
	Droplet	0.1125	0.8875		
Deboarding	Contact	0.0001	0.9999	0.0101	0.9899
	Droplet	0.0100	0.9900		

Table 4.7 Probabilities of elementary events occurring in means of collective public transport – variant 1: with masks

Event	Transmission route	P(Ai)	1-P(Ai)	P	1-P
Ticket purchase	Contact	0.0001	0.9999	0.0001	0.9999
Boarding	Contact	0.0001	0.9999	0.0040	0.9960
	Droplet	*0.0039*	0.9961		
Ticket validation	-----	-----	-----	-----	-----
Travelling	Contact	0.0001	0.9999	0.044213	0.9558
	Droplet	*0.0441*	0.9559		
Deboarding	Contact	0.0001	0.9999	0.004021	0.9960
	Droplet	*0.0039*	0.9961		

$$P(A_2 \ u \ A_3) = 1 - 0.9999*0.9961 = 0.0039996$$

$$P(A_5 \ u \ A_6) = 1 - 0.9999*0.9559 = 0.04419559$$

$$P(A_7 \ u \ A_8) = 1 - 0.9999*0.9961 = 0.0039996$$

Finally, following the relevant substitutions in formula 4.13, one could obtain the total probability for the variant in which passengers wear protective masks:

$$P = 1 - (1-0.0001)*(1-0.0039996)*(1-0.\ 04419559)*(1-0.0039996)$$
$$= 0.0519 = \textbf{5.19\%}$$

The foregoing clearly implies the difference in the probability of viral pathogen transmission between the cases when masks are not used and when masks are worn, as it comes to as much as 7.86% for the first variant, which is more than 150% of the lower value. The sources of these differences have been marked as italic font in Table 4.7.

4.4.1.3.2 Variant 2

The passenger takes a standing place having purchased the ticket via a mobile application. Compared to variant 1, in this case, the risk resulting directly from making the payment can be eliminated (Table 4.8).

4.4.1.3.3 Variant 3

The passenger takes a seat having bought the ticket at a kiosk. In this case, unlike in variant 1, the threat of touching railings and handles while travelling can be ruled out Table 4.9).

Table 4.8 Probabilities of elementary events occurring in means of collective public transport – variant 2: with and without masks

Event	Transmission route	P(Ai)	1-P(Ai)	P	1-P
Without masks					
Ticket purchase	-----	-----	-----	-----	-----
Boarding	Contact	0.0001	0.9999	0.0101	0.9899
	Droplet	0.0100	0.9900		
Ticket validation	-----	-----	-----	-----	-----
Travelling	Contact	0.0001	0.9999	0.1126	0.8874
	Droplet	0.1125	0.8875		
Deboarding	Contact	0.0001	0.9999	0.0101	0.9899
	Droplet	0.0100	0.9900		
Total probability: 0.13042 = 13.042%					
With masks					
Ticket purchase	-----	-----	-----	-----	-----
Boarding	Contact	0.0001	0.9999	0.0040	0.9960
	Droplet	0.0039	0.9961		
Ticket validation	-----	-----	-----	-----	-----
Travelling	Contact	0.0001	0.9999	0.044213	0.9558
	Droplet	0.0441	0.9559		
Deboarding	Contact	0.0001	0.9999	0.004021	0.9960
	Droplet	0.0039	0.9961		
Total probability: 0.05188 = 5.188%					

Table 4.9 Probabilities of elementary events occurring in means of collective public transport – variant 3: with and without masks

Event	Transmission route	P(Ai)	1-P(Ai)	P	1-P
Without masks					
Ticket purchase	Contact	0.0001	0.9999	0.0001	0.9999
Boarding	Contact	0.0001	0.9999	0.0101	0.9899
	Droplet	0.0100	0.9900		
Ticket validation	-----	-----	-----	-----	-----
Travelling	-----	-----	-----	0.1125	0.8875
	Droplet	0.1125	0.8875		
Deboarding	Contact	0.0001	0.9999	0.0101	0.9899
	Droplet	0.0100	0.9900		
Total probability: 0.13042 = 13.042%					
With masks					
Ticket purchase	Contact	0.0001	0.9999	0.0001	0.9999
Boarding	Contact	0.0001	0.9999	0.0040	0.9960
	Droplet	0.0039	0.9961		
Ticket validation	-----	-----	-----	-----	-----
Travelling	-----	-----	-----	0.04412	0.9559
	Droplet	0.0441	0.9559		
Deboarding	Contact	0.0001	0.9999	0.004021	0.9960
	Droplet	0.0039	0.9961		
Total probability: 0.05188 = 5.188%					

4.4.1.3.4 Variant 4

The passenger takes a seat having bought the ticket via the mobile application. Compared to variant 3, in this case, the risk resulting directly from making the payment can be eliminated (Table 4.10).

The above analyses of individual variants represent the services of collective public transport by buses, trams or trolleybuses. In order to analyse underground railway as a form of collective public transport, one should consider its specificity in terms of the confined space of its external transport infrastructure and typical forms of payment. The calculations addressing this case have been provided in the collective summary further on in this chapter.

Table 4.10 Probabilities of elementary events occurring in means of collective public transport – variant 4: with and without masks

Event	Transmission route	P(Ai)	1-P(Ai)	P	1-P
Without masks					
Ticket purchase	-----	-----	-----	-----	-----
Boarding	Contact	0.0001	0.9999	0.0101	0.9899
	Droplet	0.0100	0.9900		
Ticket validation	-----	-----	-----	-----	-----
Travelling	-----	-----	-----	0.1125	0.8875
	Droplet	0.1125	0.8875		
Deboarding	Contact	0.0001	0.9999	0.0101	0.9899
	Droplet	0.0100	0.9900		
Total probability: 0.13034 = 13.034%					
With masks					
Ticket purchase	-----	-----	-----	-----	-----
Boarding	Contact	0.0001	0.9999	0.0040	0.9960
	Droplet	0.0039	0.9961		
Ticket validation	-----	-----	-----	-----	-----
Travelling	-----	-----	-----	0.04412	0.9559
	Droplet	0.0441	0.9559		
Deboarding	Contact	0.0001	0.9999	0.004021	0.9960
	Droplet	0.0039	0.9961		
Total probability: 0.05179 = 5.179%					

4.4.2 Case Study of Car Sharing

4.4.2.1 General Assumptions

In car sharing services, persons who rent a car drive it themselves, which means that there is neither another driver nor a third person inside the vehicle. This implies that it is not possible to become infected via droplets while driving. Vehicles are disinfected after each use, which significantly reduces the possibility of touch infection. All those participating in this service, i.e., the persons renting vehicles and the rental company personnel, must wear face masks. Two variants have been taken into consideration with regard to the car sharing service, namely, vehicle rental at a customer service point (car rental desk) and at a self-service rental point.

4.4.2.2 Identification of Infection Mechanisms in Consecutive Process Steps

With reference to the map representing the car sharing service process (Chapter 3, Figure 3.4), the following activities which may involve virus transmission were defined and characterised.

Vehicle collection at a customer service point:

1 Vehicle pick-up: there is a contact with the customer service agent, but it is short – assumed to be 5 min. One is exposed to the risk of contact infection by touch when collecting keys.
2 Entering: one is exposed to the risk of infection by touching vehicle components: doors, outside and inside handles.
3 Travelling: droplet infection is not possible as the person renting the vehicle travels alone. One can become infected by touching such vehicle components as the steering wheel, seat belts, gear lever or handbrake lever. However, vehicles are being disinfected.
4 Exiting: one is exposed to the risk of infection by touching vehicle components: doors, outside and inside handles.
5 Vehicle inspection: vehicle inspection can be conducted in such a way that there is no close contact between the rental company personnel and the person renting the vehicle, which eliminates the infection risk.
6 Vehicle drop-off: there is a possibility of a short contact with the service personnel – assumed to be 5 min. Consequently, droplet infection is possible.
7 Paying: one is at risk of contact infection when paying in cash. Banknotes are not disinfected and are frequently touched; moreover, the virus can persist on banknotes for a long time. There is no such risk when payment is effected by card or phone.

Self-service rental using an application:

1 Vehicle booking: Customers book vehicles via a mobile application or a website, which involves no infection risk.
2 Entering: vehicles are not disinfected after each use, which involves the possibility of infection by touching elements such as doors, outside

handles and inside handles. The author has assumed that these elements are not touched more than once every 20 min.

3 Travelling: the customer travels alone, which is why droplet infection is not possible. One can become infected by touching such vehicle components as the steering wheel, seat belts, gear lever or handbrake lever. The author has assumed that they are touched by successive users at intervals larger than 20 min.

4 Exiting: there is a risk of infection on exiting by touching vehicle elements such as doors, inside handles and outside handles. The author has assumed that these elements are touched less frequently than once every 20 min.

5 Paying: the fare payment is cashless, without contacting other people, which eliminates the infection risk.

4.4.2.3 Analysis of the Process Scenarios (Variants)

4.4.2.3.1 Variant 1

The customer rents a car at the customer service point and pays in cash (Table 4.11).

Table 4.11 Probabilities of elementary events occurring in car sharing services – variant 1: with and without masks ·

Event	Transmission route	P(Ai)	1-P(Ai)	P	1-P
With masks					
Vehicle pick-up	Droplet	0.0011	0.9989	0.0011	0.9989
	Contact	0.00001	0.9999		
Entering	Contact	0.00000001	0.99999999	0.00000001	0.99999999
Travelling	Contact	0.00000001	0.99999999	0.00000001	0.99999999
Exiting	Contact	0.00000001	0.99999999	0.00000001	0.99999999
Vehicle inspection	-----	-----	-----	-----	-----
Vehicle drop-off	Droplet	0.0011	0.9989	0.0011	0.9989
Payment	Contact	0.0001	0.9999	0.0001	0.9999
Total probability: 0.00229 = **0.229%**					
Without masks					
Vehicle pick-up	Droplet	0.0028	0.9972	0.0028	0.9972
	Contact	0.00001	0.9999		
Entering	Contact	0.00000001	0.99999999	0.00000001	0.99999999
Travelling	Contact	0.00000001	0.99999999	0.00000001	0.99999999
Exiting	Contact	0.00000001	0.99999999	0.00000001	0.99999999
Vehicle inspection	-----	-----	-----	-----	-----
Vehicle drop-off	Droplet	0.0028	0.9972	0.0028	0.9972
Payment	Contact	0.0001	0.9999	0.0001	0.9999
Total probability: 0.00567 = **0.567%**					

4.4.2.3.2 Variant 2

The customer rents a car at the customer service point, but the payment is cashless. In this case, the payment-related risk can be eliminated (Table 4.12).

4.4.2.3.3 Variant 3

The customer rents a car by self-service using a mobile application. In this case, the risk associated with both payment and contact with the customer service personnel can be eliminated (Table 4.13).

Table 4.12 Probabilities of elementary events occurring in car sharing services – variant 2: with and without masks

Event	Transmission route	P(Ai)	1-P(Ai)	P	1-P
With masks					
Vehicle pick-up	Droplet	0.0011	0.9989	0.0011	0.9989
	Contact	0.00001	0.9999		
Entering	Contact	0.00000001	0.99999999	0.00000001	0.99999999
Travelling	Contact	0.00000001	0.99999999	0.00000001	0.99999999
Exiting	Contact	0.00000001	0.99999999	0.00000001	0.99999999
Vehicle inspection	-----	-----	-----	-----	-----
Vehicle drop-off	Droplet	0.0011	0.9989	0.0011	0.9989
Payment	-----	-----	-----	-----	-----
Total probability: 0.00219 = **0.219%**					
Without masks					
Vehicle pick-up	Droplet	0.0028	0.9972	0.0028	0.9972
	Contact	0.00001	0.9999		
Entering	Contact	0.00000001	0.99999999	0.00000001	0.99999999
Travelling	Contact	0.00000001	0.99999999	0.00000001	0.99999999
Exiting	Contact	0.00000001	0.99999999	0.00000001	0.99999999
Vehicle inspection	-----	-----	-----	-----	-----
Vehicle drop-off	Droplet	0.0028	0.9972	0.0028	0.9972
Payment	-----	-----	-----	-----	-----
Total probability: 0.00557 = **0.557%**					

Table 4.13 Probabilities of elementary events occurring in car sharing services – variant 3: with and without masks

Event	Transmission route	P(Ai)	1-P(Ai)	P	1-P
With or without mask					
Vehicle booking	-----	-----	-----	-----	-----
Entering	Contact	0.00001	0.99999	0.00001	0.99999
Travelling	Contact	0.00001	0.99999	0.00001	0.99999
Exiting	Contact	0.00001	0.99999	0.00001	0.99999
Vehicle drop-off	-----	-----	-----	-----	-----
Payment	-----	-----	-----	-----	-----
Total probability: 0.00003 = **0.003%**					

4.4.3 Case Study of Courier Parcel Delivery Services

4.4.3.1 General Assumptions

With regard to courier services, three parcel delivery options were analysed:

- collection from a parcel locker,
- delivery to an indicated address,
- collection at a pick-up point.

In all these cases, all persons participating in the service should wear face masks.

4.4.3.2 Identification of Infection Mechanisms in Consecutive Process Steps

With reference to the map representing the courier service process (Chapter 3, Figure 3.5), the following activities which may involve virus transmission were defined and characterised:

1 Order placing by the customer: orders are placed via websites or by telephone, which is why the infection risk can be ruled out.
2 Paying for the order: payment is made by bank transfer, which eliminates the risk of infection.
3 Parcel handover to the courier: the customer, i.e., the person ordering the parcel, cannot become infected during this activity. However, it is possible that the courier or other employees, like the warehouse personnel, become infected, either by droplets or by touch.
4 Parcel transport by the courier: only the courier is present in the vehicle during freight, which eliminates droplet infection. Assuming that one and the same courier uses the given vehicle, infection by touch is also impossible.
5 Parcel collection by the customer:
  a From a parcel locker: the parcel should be collected from the parcel locker within 48 h following the notification that it is available. Parcels are typically packed in cardboard or plastic. The virus can persist up to 72 h on plastic surfaces, and up to 24 h on paper surfaces. This entails the risk of infection by touching the parcel itself. The parcel has been touched by the courier and the warehouse worker, which makes it a surface touched rather infrequently. Additionally, in order to collect the parcel from the parcel locker, one must enter a code using a touch screen, which also involves the possibility of infection by fomite touching. Parcel

collection from the parcel locker does not require any contact with another person, which rules out droplet infection.

b From the courier at the delivery address: droplet infection is possible, but the customer-courier contact is short. One can also maintain a safe distance, and the parcel does not have to be handed over directly from person to person. Collecting the parcel outdoors is possible, and actually practised, which also minimises the possibility of infection. The assumed time of contact with the courier is 2 min. A signature confirming the parcel receipt is not required. One can become infected by touching the parcel itself, which has been touched by the courier.

c At the pick-up point: parcel pick-up points are typically located in kiosks or stores, and so to collect the parcel one must contact the store personnel, whereupon contact with other customers is also possible. Consequently, potential droplet infection must be taken into account. The contact time is short – assumed to be 5 min. One can also become infected by touch, since the parcel being picked up has been touched by the courier and the pick-up point personnel.

4.4.3.3 Analysis of the Process Scenarios (Variants)

4.4.3.3.1 Variant I

Courier service involving parcel collection at a pick-up point with customer service (Table 4.14).

Table 4.14 Probabilities of elementary events associated with the courier service – variant I: with and without masks

Event	Transmission route	P(Ai)	I-P(Ai)
With masks			
Order placing	-----	-----	-----
Payment	-----	-----	-----
Parcel handover to the courier	-----	-----	-----
Parcel shipment	-----	-----	-----
Parcel collection	Droplet	0.00001	0.9999
	Contact	0.0049	0.9951
Total probability: 0.00491 = 0.491%			
Without masks			
Order placing	-----	-----	-----
Payment	-----	-----	-----
Parcel handover to the courier	-----	-----	-----
Parcel shipment	-----	-----	-----
Parcel collection	Droplet	0.00001	0.9999
	Contact	0.0125	0.9875
Total probability: 0.01251 = 1.251%			

4.4.3.3.2 Variant 2

Courier service involving parcel delivery to a specific address and personal collection (Table 4.15).

4.4.3.3.3 Variant 3

Courier service involving parcel collection from a parcel locker. There is no direct contact in this variant, which makes it irrelevant whether or not masks are worn (Table 4.16).

Table 4.15 Probabilities of elementary events associated with the courier service – variant 2: with and without masks

Event	Transmission route	P(Ai)	I-P(Ai)
With masks			
Order placing	-----	-----	-----
Payment	-----	-----	-----
Parcel handover to the courier	-----	-----	-----
Parcel shipment	-----	-----	-----
Parcel collection	Droplet	0.00001	0.9999
	Contact	0.001961	0.998039
Total probability: 0.00197 = 0.197%			
Without masks			
Order placing	-----	-----	-----
Payment	-----	-----	-----
Parcel handover to the courier	-----	-----	-----
Parcel shipment	-----	-----	-----
Parcel collection	Droplet	0.00001	0.9999
	Contact	0.005	0.995
Total probability: 0.00501 = 0.501%			

Table 4.16 Probabilities of elementary events associated with the courier service – variant 2: with and without masks

Event	Transmission route	P(Ai)	I-P(Ai)
With or without masks			
Order placing	-----	-----	-----
Payment	-----	-----	-----
Parcel handover to the courier	-----	-----	-----
Parcel shipment	-----	-----	-----
Parcel collection	Droplet	0.00001	0.9999
	Contact	0.00001	0.99999
Total probability: 0.00011 = 0.011%			

4.5 DISCUSSION

As described above, further detailed analyses were conducted and probabilities of elementary events were determined, and on such basis the total probabilities of viral pathogen transmission were calculated for other transport services.

On account of the different configurations of elementary events involving the probability of virus transmission, several implementation options were adopted for each of the services.

The following variants were analysed for the remaining transport services, all of which included alternatives with and without masks:

1 Rail transport – long-distance train:
   a ticket purchase at a ticket office or from a ticket machine, and personal ticket inspection during the travel
   b ticket purchase using an application and personal ticket inspection during the travel
2 Air transport:
   a travelling without checked luggage and without bus transport to and from the airport apron
   b travelling without checked luggage, with bus transport only to or only from the airport apron
   c travelling without checked luggage, with bus transport both to and from the airport apron
   d travelling with checked luggage, without bus transport to and from the airport apron
   e travelling with checked luggage, with bus transport only to or only from the airport apron
   f travelling with checked luggage, with bus transport both to and from the airport apron
3 Underground railway:
   a a passenger takes a standing place having purchased the ticket from a ticket machine (considering the period of waiting on the platform perceived as a confined space as well as entering and exiting the metro station)
   b a passenger using a smart card takes a standing place (considering the period of waiting on the platform perceived as a confined space as well as entering and exiting the metro station)
   c a passenger takes a seat having purchased the ticket from a ticket machine (considering the period of waiting on the platform perceived as a confined space as well as entering and exiting the metro station)
   d a passenger using a smart card takes a seat (considering the period of waiting on the platform perceived as a confined space as well as entering and exiting the metro station)

4 Regular service (intercity) coaches:
   a a passenger takes a seat having purchased the ticket using an application
   b a passenger takes a seat having purchase the ticket from the driver or at the service desk,
5 Individual transport – taxi:
   a travel and payment in cash
   b travel and cashless payment (using an application)
6 Food delivery (catering):
   a payment in cash,
   b cashless payment,
7 Grocery delivery:
   a payment in cash
   b cashless payment
8 Heavy transport (over 3.5 tonnes):
   a unloading with the driver involved
   b unloading without the driver involved.

In accordance with the algorithm assumed in the methodology proposed for calculating the probability of viral pathogen transmission (Figure 4.4), the values of total probability have been determined for the performance of the above transport services under specific variants, as summarised in Table 4.17. The numbers of individual variants are analogical to the sequence in which they have been stated in the previous paragraph. The above letter designations of sub-items, i.e. (a), (b), etc., indicate successive variants 1, 2, etc. in the table, and address the consecutive types of transport services (e.g. "Taxi, variant 1 – mask" corresponds to item 5 above, i.e. Individual transport – taxi: a) travel and payment in cash). With regard to the services of collective urban transport, car sharing and courier parcel delivery, described in detail in the previous section, the variant numbers correspond to those provided in the description.

For purposes of a comparative analysis of the transport services in question, statistical parameters of the distribution of the values obtained were determined, namely, the median, standard deviation and extreme values, for the variants involving the highest and the lowest probability of viral pathogen transmission.

A collective summary of these parameters is provided in Table 4.18.

The foregoing makes it possible to rank individual passenger and freight transport services, from those which involve the lowest probability of viral pathogen transmission to those where it is most likely. This ranking is illustrated Figures 4.7 and 4.8. They imply that, in terms of viral infection, the safest passenger transport service is car sharing, while the service entailing the highest threat is long-distance regular coach service. Under the category of freight transport, the differences between individual variants

Table 4.17 Summary of total probabilities for all transport services broken down into several variants, with and without masks

Service variant	Variant 1		Variant 2		Variant 3		Variant 4		Variant 5		Variant 6	
	Mask	No mask	Mask	No mask	Mask	No mask	Mask	No mask	Mask	No mask	Mask	No mask
Probability	p [%]	p [%]	p [%]	p [%]	p [%]	p [%]	p [%]	p [%]	p [%]	p [%]	p [%]	p [%]
Transport service	**Passenger transport**											
Collective urban transport	5.198	13.051	5.188	13.042	5.188	13.042	5.179	13.034				
Taxi	0.337	0.842	0.327	0.832								
Car sharing	0.229	0.567	0.219	0.557	0.003	0.003						
Regular coach service	16.363	41.212	16.699	41.800								
Underground railway	3.252	8.042	3.243	8.033	3.243	8.033	3.233	8.024				
Railway transport	12.034	30.147	12.025	30.140								
Air transport	9.200	22.643	10.267	24.948	11.321	27.184	9.646	23.611	10.707	25.887	11.757	28.095
Courier parcel delivery services	**Freight transport**											
Courier parcel delivery services	0.011	0.011	0.197	0.501	0.491	1.251						
Food delivery (catering)	0.207	0.511	0.197	0.501								
Grocery delivery	0.207	0.511	0.197	0.501								
Heavy transport	1.472	3.751	0.001	0.001								

Table 4.18 Statistics and ranking of the probabilities of viral pathogen transmission for different transport services

Statistics	Median	STD	Variant max.	Variant min.
Probability	p [%]	p [%]	p [%]	p [%]
Transport service	**Passenger transport**			
Car sharing	0.224	0.230	0.567	0.003
Taxi	0.585	0.252	0.842	0.327
Underground railway	5.638	2.395	8.042	3.233
Collective urban transport	9.116	3.927	13.051	5.179
Air transport	17.200	7.603	28.095	9.200
Railway transport	21.087	9.057	30.147	12.025
Regular coach service	28.955	12.490	41.800	16.363
	Freight transport			
Courier parcel delivery services	0.344	0.425	1.251	0.011
Food delivery (catering)	0.354	0.152	0.511	0.197
Grocery delivery	0.354	0.152	0.511	0.197
Heavy transport	0.736	1.534	3.751	0.001

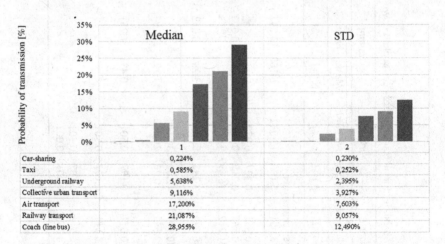

Figure 4.7 Comparison of mean viral pathogen transmission probability values, including standard deviation, for passenger transport services.

analysed are much smaller, and the service with the highest calculated viral pathogen transmission probability is heavy transport. This result may be surprising, but it is directly linked with another observation which clearly stems from the results obtained, namely, that the factor which exerts by far the greatest impact on the value of the probability of viral pathogen transmission in transport services is the time of exposure to the pathogen in

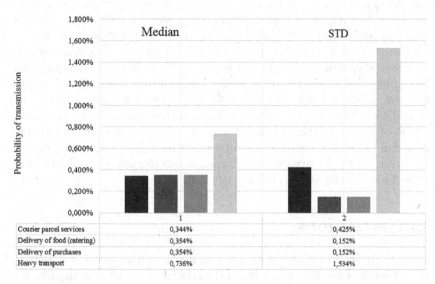

	Median	STD
Courier parcel services	0,344%	0,425%
Delivery of food (catering)	0,354%	0,152%
Delivery of purchases	0,354%	0,152%
Heavy transport	0,736%	1,534%

Figure 4.8 Comparison of mean viral pathogen transmission probability values, including standard deviation, for freight transport services.

Table 4.19 Total probabilities of viral pathogen transmission and overall infection probability in transport services with reference to the factor of active disease cases

Probability	Total	Overall
Transport service	*p [%]*	*p [%]*
Passenger transport		
Car sharing	0.224	**0.0022**[a]
Taxi	0.585	**0.0058**
Underground railway	5.638	**0.0563**
Collective urban transport	9.116	**0.0912**
Air transport	17.200	**0.1720**
Railway transport	21.087	**0.2109**
Regular coach service	28.955	**0.2896**
Freight transport		
Courier parcel delivery services	0.344	**0.0034**
Food delivery (catering)	0.354	**0.0035**
Grocery delivery	0.354	**0.0035**
Heavy transport	0.736	**0.0074**

Note:
[a] Bold values represent the overall probability of infection in transport service with assumption of IFR of epidemic.

interpersonal contacts. In the case of heavy transport, the driver's involvement in unloading and the subsequent contact with the end customer results in higher probability values compared to other freight transport services.

In order to determine the overall probability of viral infection attributable to the provision of transport services, the probability resulting from the number of active infections across the population must be taken into account. Moreover, according to estimates referred to above, this figure should be adjusted by considering active undiagnosed cases (conversion factor of 5). As of the end of November 2020, the ratio of the number of active COVID-19 cases to the total population of Poland was 0.622%. However, taking the dynamic of the epidemic development trend, this ratio should be assumed as 1% (Table 4.19).

4.6 CONCLUSIONS

It is very difficult to calculate the probability of viral infection in transport, which results from the specificity of the related processes conditioning the number of random events involving the probability of activating a virus transmission mechanism (via droplets, by touching a contaminated surface or in direct contact with a potentially sick person). The virus transmission models proposed to date, even if dedicated to specific means of transport, are actually limited to droplet transmission in spaces corresponding to individual means of transport. Since transport processes comprise an abundance of such events which may involve virus transmission by touch, a different approach to the problem in question has been proposed. Obviously, in terms of absolute values and from the perspective of the likelihood of effective virus transmission, the droplet mechanism is definitely the predominant one, yet the number of events involving the remaining transmission mechanisms and their relation with the daily scale of provision of all transport services cause that even seemingly small differences, ranging at tenths or even hundredths of per cent, trigger serious quantitative effects. The next chapter of this monograph is entirely devoted to this problem.

Considering all the foregoing observations, the author of this monograph decided to develop a universal methodology for estimating the probability of viral pathogen transmission by referring to the SARS-CoV-2 pandemic, assuming full mathematical disclosure and an open process formula, aimed to make it possible to take specific other mechanisms of virus transmission into account when providing transport services. When calculating the total probability of viral pathogen transmission in the given transport service, the author referred to the definition of probability of a sum of independent events. The presentng values are not the value of the probability of infection, but the value of the probability of transmission of the pathogen, assuming that the pathogen is in the means of transport. There is still a very random path from the transmission of the pathogen to the infection (taking into account the amount of the pathogen, the resistance of the organism, age, etc.) and here a separate probability calculation would have to be made.

Total probability of viral pathogen transmission represents an average value from several variants and for different situations (for passenfger transport: including taking a seat on the mean of transport and the distance from the infected person). Equally well, assuming 100% disinfection, that everyone wears N95, KN95 or FFP3 masks correctly, avoids touching the surface, there is only one person infected with very low pathogen spread ratio the probability then may be minimal.

Of course, this probability is distributed differently among passengers and depends on the seat and distance from the infected person, on the behavior of people (the infected and exposed), etc. This is a value averaged over several different variants of the journey and all passengers, including extreme cases: one person sits next to the infected one and the other at the other end of the mean of transport.

Chapter 5

Methodology for Estimating the Exposure to and Effects of Viral Infection in Transport Services

5.1 PRINCIPLES OF THE METHODOLOGY FOR ESTIMATING THE EXPOSURE TO AND EFFECTS OF VIRAL INFECTION IN TRANSPORT SERVICES

Risk assessment requires not only estimation of the probability that an adverse event occurs, to which studies and analyses of transport-related risk are typically limited, but also estimation of the exposure to and consequences of that event. Exposure to an adverse event, depending on its type, can be understood as the exposure which one can express in terms of the intensity of the given phenomenon or the exposure duration. With regard to the epidemic risk analysis for transport services, exposure time was adopted as the measure of exposure, which was assumed to ensure unambiguousness of interpretation by the user of the method proposed and simplicity of the algorithm applied to estimate this value. A significantly more difficult challenge is assessing the effects of exposure to an adverse event. Many risk assessment methods refer to the notion of damage to health as a measure of these effects, including serious health consequences and fatalities. Given the assumed universal nature of the method developed by the author for purposes of assessment of the epidemic risk (viral infection) associated with transport, which in this case is represented by the SARS-CoV-2 pandemic, and considering the incomplete nature of the knowledge of the consequences of COVID-19, it was decided that the effects of occurrence of an adverse event would be estimated as the number of fatalities nationwide.

No knowledge about the sources of infection, particularly in transport services, is currently available. Although there are pandemic control strategies which assume identification and containment of outbreaks, the source (outbreak) of infection in transport services is virtually never defined (with the exception of public transport). The lack of such knowledge significantly hinders estimation of the effects of the coronavirus infection in transport services. That is precisely why the author decided to develop a complete methodology for estimating the fatality rate attributable to the

DOI: 10.1201/9781003204732-5

SARS-CoV-2 infection for different transport services based on statistical methods.

For this purpose, an extensive study and review of the current state of knowledge on the spread of the SARS-CoV-2 virus and the effects of COVID-19 was conducted by referring to the example of Poland. They were followed by statistical analyses of the Polish transport sector. Another step was developing transport service models based on the process maps previously designed (Chapter 3), which were prepared for the purpose of identification of the hazard factors typical of transport services according to the Deep Hazard Identification (DHI) method. This made it possible to estimate chains of events and contact activities involving the probability of virus transmission. This methodology enabled the author to estimate the number of people at risk of infection while participating in a transport service. Additionally, the numbers of exposed persons determined in this manner were adjusted by the share factor in a breakdown into specific age groups, given the considerable age-related differences in terms of COVID-19-related fatality rate.

The data thus obtained made it possible to estimate the effects of infection expressed as the average number of fatalities against the given group of transport services.

In order to compare different types of services in passenger and freight transport, some cumulative indicators were assumed as representative of the nationwide effects. This assumption adds value to the methodology in question, making it applicable to strategic analyses of pandemic control on a national policy scale.

5.2 METHOD FOR DETERMINING INDICATORS OF THE EFFECTS OF VIRAL INFECTION IN TRANSPORT SERVICES

In the initial phase of implementation of the method in question, one should determine sets of relevant indicators enabling quantitative estimation. These indicators are based on statistical measures representing specific data sets. This makes it possible to extrapolate the results obtained for a specific sample (event) based on representative statistical measures. In the absence of direct source data on the SARS-CoV-2 infections and fatalities associated with transport services, the methodology proposed by the author enables the relevant quantities to be estimated.

With reference to the analysis of the available medical knowledge on the SARS-CoV-2 epidemic, it was established undoubtedly that the effects of COVID-19 are highly dependent on the age of the sick person.

Most studies conducted in this field are based on analysis of unit data concerning infected persons. The updated analyses performed by a team representing the Faculty of Mathematics, Informatics and Mechanics of the University of Warsaw by application of the competing risks method (Ghani et al., 2005; Fine and Gray, 1999), being a generalised version of the classical Kaplan–Meier methods of survival analysis, translated into a situation where the patient's condition at the end of observation is described by more than two states. According to this method, the survival analysis technique is based on estimation of the product limit, as proposed by Kaplan and Meier in 1958 (Brok, 1998). The method makes it possible to plot a cumulative distribution of survival, estimate the probability of survival and establish the risk of death. The Kaplan–Meier estimator (Kaplan et al., 1958) is a non-parametric statistic used to estimate the survival function from lifetime data, and it is given by:

$$\hat{S}(t) = \prod_{i:t_i \leq t}\left(1 - \frac{d_i}{n_i}\right) \tag{5.1}$$

where:

t_i – time when at least one event happened,
d_i – number of events (e.g. deaths) that happened at time t_i,
n_i – individuals known to have survived up to time t_i.

The Kaplan–Meier estimator is currently used in many studies and analyses of COVID-19-related mortality (Beigel et al., 2020; Sousa et al., 2020; Goshua et al., 2020).

In the studies addressed in the Faculty of Mathematics, Informatics and Mechanics of the University of Warsaw with regard to COVID-19, using the competing risks method, death, recovery or absence of either of these two events were defined as events. The case fatality rate (CFR) estimate is obtained by considering the probability of both death and recovery, as given by the following equation:

$$CFR = \frac{\theta_0}{(\theta_0 - \theta_1)} \tag{5.2}$$

where:

θ_0 – probability of death,
θ_1 – probability of recovery within a period of time from the diagnosis to the maximum observation time.

As indicated by the preceding analyses by researchers from the University of Warsaw, the case fatality rate in the age group of 66–75 years in Poland was 12.43 times higher (95% confidence interval [CI]: 9.47–16.32), and in the 76+ years age group it was 25.68 times higher (95% CI: 20.12–32.78) than in the age group of 0–65 years, which is consistent with observations from other countries. Similarly, the fatality rate is higher among men than among women (hazard ratios (HR) 1.61, 95% CI 1.33–1.95). Similar results have been presented in Russell et al. (2020) with reference to estimation of the infection and case fatality rate for COVID-19 using age-adjusted data from the outbreak on the Diamond Princess cruise ship.

The general health condition and the concomitant diseases have obviously also a significant impact on the course of COVID-19. However, since it was impossible to obtain a data set describing the health condition of the persons participating in transport processes, and at the same time, it is a common approach, even in medicine, to assume that the general health condition is statistically represented by a specific age group, this particular breakdown was adopted as the first indicator. The foregoing approach was additionally substantiated by the higher accessibility of data sets thus segregated, for example, in studies concerning collective public transport. Studies based on comprehensive traffic surveys addressing the problems of urban mobility and public transport break down the population into specific age groups. On account of the breakdown of the transport process participants by age group, it was necessary to divide the age ranges further on in order to match the relevant mobility characteristics. This assumption made it difficult to apply the Kaplan–Meier estimators, and hence the need for dedicated coefficients.

Therefore, precisely based on these age categories, the method in question adopted the following breakdown into age groups of the persons participating in the processes associated with the provision of the chosen transport services:

- children – age ranging between 0 and 14 years,
- young people and students – age ranging between 15 and 24 years,
- working age, young workers – age ranging between 25 and 44 years,
- working age, older workers – age ranging between 45 and 64 years,
- retirement age (active in terms of mobility) – age ranging between 65 and 84 years,
- late retirement age (passive in terms of mobility) – age of 85 years and more.

Given the above assumptions, the case fatality rate was estimated by analysing the publicly available data on infections and deaths on consecutive days of the epidemic. The case fatality rate on consecutive days of the epidemic was estimated by dividing the cumulative number of fatalities on a given day by the cumulative number of cases on the same day.

Another important indicator was the COVID-19 mortality factor (M_f), given by the following relationship:

$$M_f = \frac{M}{P} \tag{5.3}$$

where:

M – number of fatalities attributable to COVID-19 in the given country,
P – population of the country.

With regard to COVID-19, the mortality factor is strongly dependent on age. Therefore, for purposes of the method in question, it was proposed that the mortality factors should be computed for each of the predefined age groups separately, according to the following formula:

$$M_{fa} = \frac{M_a}{P_a} \tag{5.4}$$

where:

M_a – number of fatalities attributable to COVID-19 in a specific age group in the given country,
P_a – population of a specific age group in the given country.

About 8 months after the first diagnosed case of the SARS-CoV-2 infection, i.e. on 4 November 2020, the following figures were reported in the USA (Table 5.1).

Table 5.1 Size of age groups and number of fatalities attributable to COVID-19 in USA (as of 4 November 2020)

Age group (years)	Number of fatalities	Population	Share of fatalities (%)
0–14	79	60,570,846	0.00013
15–24	400	42,687,510	0.00094
25–44	6,010	87,599,465	0.0069
45–64	39,045	83,323,439	0.047
65–84	104,854	47,453,305	0.22
85+	66,960	6,604,958	1.01

Table 5.2 COVID-19 mortality factors by age group

Age group (years)	Mortality factor – M_{fa}
0–14	0.0000013
15–24	0.0000094
25–44	0.000069
45–64	0.00047
65–84	0.0022
85+	0.0101

Consequently, the following age-specific mortality factors were established (Table 5.2):

Having determined the average age group share for a specific group of transport services and knowing the mortality factor (as provided in the table above), one can establish the total mortality factor (mortality indicator). The mortality factor is a representative statistical measure of the number of potential fatalities among those participating in a transport process nationwide. Once the share of individual age groups has been taken into account, the mortality indicator is calculated from the formula below:

$$M_i = \sum_{i=1}^{n} O_{ai} \cdot M_{fai} \qquad (5.5)$$

where:

O_{ai} – average share of the age group in the population participating in a transport process,

M_{fai} – mortality factor established for a specific age group (see Table 5.2),

n – number of age groups involved in the analysed transport service.

The ultimate figure expressing the number of potential fatalities among the persons who have become infected with the SARS-CoV-2 virus while participating in a transport process must obviously be correlated with the current daily rate of active cases of coronavirus-infected persons in the population, which represents the probability of a person who may be a source of virus transmission participating in the transport process.

Unfortunately, in the case of the SARS-CoV-2 virus, the course of infection, which is asymptomatic in many cases, and the time of the virus incubation in the human body, which may take even up to 14 days, make it very difficult to unambiguously determine the number of active cases (persons infected with the coronavirus) in the population. The only explicit source of knowledge in this regard is the number of positive tests for viral infection, accumulated and corrected by the number of people who have recovered or, unfortunately, died. Such a measure is the number of active cases. However, one should take the actual numbers of active cases into consideration. Experts estimate that the actual number may be more than five times higher than that reported by health care organisations or governmental institutions due to the small number of tests as well as some behaviour patterns of people who deliberately avoid being tested despite the symptoms of infection or those who are asymptomatic. Scientists from the Faculty of Mathematics, Informatics and Mechanics of the University of Warsaw established an accurate value based on the median value of the ratio of people diagnosed daily to the daily number of all infected persons, which is a multiple of 5.6 persons.

With regard to the foregoing, the following formula for determining the daily indicator of active SARS-CoV-2 infection cases was adopted for purposes of the methodology in question:

$$I_a = \frac{I \cdot (n-1)}{P} \qquad (5.6)$$

where:

I – officially reported daily number of cases (of the disease in question) in the given country,

n – multiple representing the non-reported daily number of cases in the given country,

P – population of the country.

Analysing the Polish sector of transport services, and referring to some expert opinions of epidemiologists, the n coefficient (multiple representing the non-reported daily number of cases in a given country) was assumed to be equal to 5. The $(n-1)$ component of the formula results from an assumption that the persons who have been positively diagnosed for coronavirus remain in compulsory quarantine and do not participate in transport processes, neither as customer nor as employees. The distribution of the values of the daily indicator of active SARS-CoV-2 infection cases thus calculated by Equation 5.6 for Poland since the onset of the pandemic is presented in Figure 5.1.

As the Figure 5.1 implies, the value of this indicator is highly variable, with a particularly dynamic increase observed at the end of September, which was due to the severity of the pandemic in Poland in this period. On account of such high variability, assuming a mean value from the entire history of the SARS-CoV-2 epidemic in Poland with regard to a single period

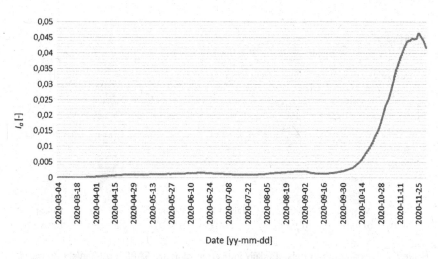

Figure 5.1 Distribution of Poland's daily indicators of active SARS-CoV-2 infection cases.

of time would be encumbered with a considerable error. Therefore, it is recommended that one should assume values based on an analysis of trend and recurrence at individual stages of the epidemic. In order to illustrate this phenomenon, scenario analyses were performed for six variants:

1 for nine randomly selected days, each one in a consecutive month of the epidemic,
2 for one day in the peak month of the pandemic in Poland (the highest number of fatalities of 674 was reported on 25 November),
3 for averaged values from the first month of the pandemic in Poland (March 2020),
4 for averaged values from August, being a holiday month in Poland, when the infection curve was observed to have flattened,
5 for averaged values from November, being the peak month of the pandemic in Poland (with top infection and fatality figures),
6 for averaged values for the period from the first diagnosed SARS-CoV-2 infection in Poland until 30 November 2020.

The indicators of active SARS-CoV-2 infection cases calculated for the above variants are provided in Table 5.3 and Figure 5.2.

Table 5.3 Indicators of active SARS-CoV-2 infection cases for variants 1–6

	Variant 1	Variant 2	Variant 3	Variant 4	Variant 5	Variant 6
I_a	0.0072111	0.0463426	0.0000612	0.0016128	0.0392069	0.0061507

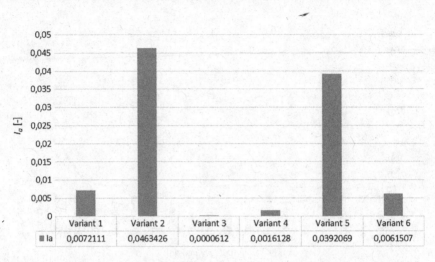

	Variant 1	Variant 2	Variant 3	Variant 4	Variant 5	Variant 6
■ Ia	0,0072111	0,0463426	0,0000612	0,0016128	0,0392069	0,0061507

Figure 5.2 Distribution of Poland's daily indicators of active SARS-CoV-2 infection cases.

5.3 ESTIMATION OF FATALITY RATES ATTRIBUTABLE TO VIRAL INFECTION IN TRANSPORT AS A MEASURE OF THE EFFECTS OF EPIDEMIC THREATS

In order to assess the extent and effects of the epidemic threats in transport, one should also consider the number of persons exposed to viral infection. Due to the specific nature of the provision of transport services, especially in a breakdown into passenger and freight transport services, each service type requires a different approach. For passenger transport, the value in question corresponds to the number of passengers and drivers (transport operators) or, if necessary, the number of persons in the service personnel. For the freight transport sector, one must establish the number of persons involved in a chain of events comprising the activities which involve interpersonal contact in the process and the number of customers in the case of self-collection. What proves to be particularly useful when identifying the contact activities in the chain of events and the persons participating in passenger transport is the process maps presented in Chapter 3.

In this case, it is very important not to treat the number of exposed persons as a definite and final value. This is due to the specificity of the effects of the epidemic threat, namely, COVID-19 case fatality rate. As mentioned before, the mortality factor for this hazard is strongly age dependent. Therefore, one should adjust the exposure assessment by mortality indicator M_i (Equation 5.5) having considered the share of age groups (O_a) and the mortality factors established separately for each of the predefined age groups (M_{fa}) (Equation 5.4).

The ultimate measure of the effects of epidemic threats in transport services is the total fatality rate due to viral infection. Based on the coefficients thus determined, one can estimate the case fatality rate in a specific group of transport services as the potential total number of persons who have died due to being infected with the SARS-CoV-2 virus while participating in a transport process. This quantity should be assumed as the consequence in the risk assessment. The total mortality rate value is determined by the following formula:

$$M_t = L \cdot M_i \cdot I_a \tag{5.7}$$

where:

   L – number of participants in the transport process exposed to viral infection,

   M_i – mortality indicator taking the share of age groups into account,

   I_a – indicator of active SARS-CoV-2 infection cases in the given country.

5.4 ESTIMATING THE NUMBER OF PERSONS EXPOSED TO VIRAL INFECTION IN TRANSPORT AND TOTAL FATALITY RATES

The author has proposed dedicated methods for estimating the number of persons exposed to viral infection in transport, which are universal in nature but which require analysis of the specifics of the given transport service.

In order to illustrate the method, two examples of statistical estimation of the number of persons exposed to viral infection are presented – one for passenger transport and the other for freight transport.

Collective public transport was chosen as an example of a service delivered in the passenger transport sector, since on account of its predominant quantitative share, it is by far the most relevant one for the analysis of epidemic threats in transport.

Firstly, based on the results of periodic comprehensive traffic surveys, the percentage share of individual age groups in the passenger structure should be established. Sample results of actual daily values obtained for three large agglomerations are provided in Table 5.4.

After compiling large sets of publicly available data provided in reports on comprehensive traffic surveys, mean values of the share of passengers participating in collective public transport were established in a breakdown into age groups, which made it possible to determine the mean values of the M_{fa} mortality factor for specific age groups (Equation 5.4) and of the M_i total mortality indicator of collective public transport (Equation 5.5). The values thus established are summarised in Table 5.5.

Table 5.4 Daily values of the share of passengers in collective public transport by age groups

Age group (years)	Agglomeration 1		Agglomeration 2		Agglomeration 3	
	No. of passengers	Percentage share (%)	No. of passengers	Percentage share (%)	No. of passengers	Percentage share (%)
up to 14	28,773	5.1	23,712	20.4	89,356	7.9
15–24	106,951	18.9	35,053	30.1	285,517	25.4
25–44	177,557	31.3	30,929	26.5	299,698	26.6
55–64	130,991	23.1	17,733	15.2	278,072	24.7
65–84	122,851	21.7	9,073	7.8	173,384	15.4
85+						
TOTAL	567,123	100	116,500	100	1,126,027	100

Table 5.5 Age-specific mortality factors and total mortality indicator for collective public transport

Age group (years)	O_a (%)	M_{fa}	M_i	M_i (%)
Up to 15	11.1	0.0000013	0.000000145	0.000015
16–24	24.8	0.0000094	0.000002321	0.00023
25–44	28.2	0.000069	0.000019318	0.0019
45–64	21.0	0.00047	0.000098426	0.0098
65–84	14.9	0.0032	0.000475133	0.048
85+				
TOTAL	100	0.0037262	**0.000595**	**0.060**

As provided in statistics and reports on the Polish transport sector, 5,294,384 passengers used collective public transport each day in 2019. Given the significant declines observed in the figures characterising the passenger transport sector during the pandemic and the restrictions (interventions) imposed on public transport, defining the admissible occupancy of the means of transport at 50% (30%) of the permissible number of passengers, it was found that the number of passengers dropped by as much as 70% (Table 5.6 and Figure 5.3).

Therefore, the mean daily volume of passengers transported by collective public services in Poland during the pandemic is ca. 1,588,315 passengers. The total mortality rate values determined by formula 5.7 for the assumed variants are provided in Table 5.7.

An analogical estimation was performed for a sample service delivered in the freight transport sector. On account of its relevance for the overall assessment of the epidemic hazard vis-à-vis transport at large, an analysis of the courier parcel delivery service sector has been provided as an example.

Table 5.6 Quantitative year-over-year comparison of road passenger transport figures
for corresponding periods including the pandemic in Poland

Passenger transport (road) ('000)

Year	III	IV	V	VI	VII	VIII	IX
2019	25,015	24,561	24,531	21,738	13301	13,556	23,866
2,020	14,338	5,331	4,986	6,884	7,061	8,246	17,236
2019	100%	100%	100%	100%	100%	100%	100%
2020	57%	22%	20%	32%	53%	61%	72%

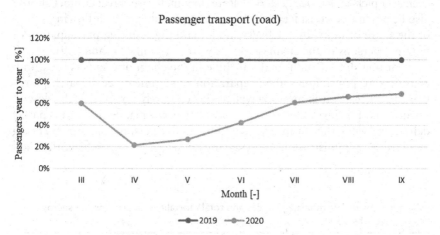

Figure 5.3 Declining percentage figures of road passenger transport due to the pandemic
as compared with the year 2019 in Poland.

Table 5.7 Total mortality rate M_t determined for public transport variants 1–6 on a
nationwide scale

	Variant 1	Variant 2	Variant 3	Variant 4	Variant 5	Variant 6
L	1,588,315					
M_i	0.000595					
I_a	0.0072111	0.0463426	0.0000612	0.0016128	0.0392069	0.0061507
M_t	*6.8148*	*43.7959*	*0.0578*	*1.5242*	*37.0524*	*5.8127*

Based on a case study, the statistical share of individual age groups in the
chain of events taking place in the provision of the relevant transport services was determined, taking into account the age of the parcel sorting office
personnel, couriers and customers involved in direct delivery. This made

it possible to estimate the mortality factors for a specific age group and the total mortality indicator for courier services. The calculation results are summarised in Table 5.8.

In order to estimate the number of persons exposed to infections in connection with courier parcel delivery services, one must consider the specifics of this service. On average, a courier delivers 35 parcels during one work shift. Some of them are delivered to parcel lockers, where direct contact between the courier and the customer is eliminated. But some are delivered directly to specific addresses, which involves direct interpersonal contact and increases the number of persons exposed (in the chain of activities). There is also a possibility to deliver the parcel to a collection point, such as a pick-up service desk or a store, in which case direct contact should also be taken into consideration. Based on a case study, the following values of the share of individual delivery modes and the resulting participation of different persons in the chain of events were determined (Table 5.9).

What one should additionally include in the chain of events is the group of people responsible for the preparation of shipments at dispatch points (sorting offices, warehouses) as well as those directly involved in the flow of documents. Having analysed the process of performance of courier parcel delivery services, the author found additional five persons, on average, being involved in administration and preparation activities. Therefore, the total

Table 5.8 Age-specific mortality factors and total mortality indicator for the sector of courier services

Age group (years)	O_a (%)	M_{fa}	M_i	M_i (%)
Up to 14	0.0	0.0000013	0.00	0.0
15–24	46.9	0.0000094	0.000004395	0.00044
25–44	51.0	0.000069	0.0000350	0.0035
45–64	2.0	0.00047	0.0000094	0.0009
65–84	0.1	0.0022	0.000002	0.00022
85+	0.0	0.0101	0.00	0.0
TOTAL	100	0.0128953	0.000051	0.0051

Table 5.9 Share of different delivery modes in the sector of courier parcel delivery services

Delivery service type	Share (%)	No. of parcels	No. of persons
Parcel locker	32	11.2	0
Direct delivery	45	15.8	17
Customer service pick-up point	23	8	9
TOTAL	100	35	26

Table 5.10 Number of deliveries and exposed persons involved in courier services per
annum and per day

A	B	C
Number of deliveries per annum ['000,000]	Number of courier deliveries per annum (A/35) ['000,000]	Number of persons exposed per annum (B*31) ['000,000]
308.1	8.803	272.886
Number of deliveries per day ['000]	Number of courier deliveries per day ['000]	Number L of persons exposed per day ['000]
844.110	24.117	747.640

Table 5.11 Total mortality rate M_t determined for courier parcel delivery service variants
1–6 on a nationwide scale

	Variant 1	Variant 2	Variant 3	Variant 4	Variant 5	Variant 6
L	747,640					
M_i	0.000051					
I_a	0.0072111	0.0463426	0.0000612	0.0016128	0.0392069	0.0061507
M_t	0.275	1.767	0.002	0.061	1.495	0.235

number of persons exposed to the related epidemic threat in the chain of
events for a single courier over one workday is 31 persons (26+5).

Based on reports on activities performed in the sector of courier parcel
delivery services in Poland, assuming the participation of 31 persons exposed
to infection in the chain of events throughout one workday of one courier,
the total average daily number of persons exposed on the nationwide scale
was estimated. The calculation results are provided in Table 5.10.

The total mortality rate values determined by formula 5.7 for the assumed
variants are presented in Table 5.11.

Statistical estimation combined with modelling of the chain of interpersonal contact events was performed analogically for the remaining transport
services. The results thus obtained are provided further on in this chapter.

5.5 ESTIMATING THE EXPOSURE AND EFFECTS OF EPIDEMIC THREATS IN TRANSPORT SERVICES

In order to estimate the number of persons exposed to and the effects (total
mortality rate) of the SARS-CoV-2 virus infection in other passenger transport services, they were grouped into collective organised and unorganised
transport (regular services) as well as individual transport (taxi and car
sharing).

The organised collective transport includes employees and school transport. On account of the current epidemic situation, school education is provided almost exclusively on a remote basis (online classes). Therefore, only employee transport was taken into consideration in the analysis. Based on reports on transport operations, it was established that the daily number of passengers using employee transport in Poland is 78,868.

The next category of services comprises regular long-distance transport, including regular coach and rail transport as well as air transport. Compared to the previous year, very significant declines in the passenger numbers were also observed in these categories due to the epidemic situation and the restrictions imposed. Coach transport suffered decreases of up to 60%, which came to ca. 35% in rail transport. The pandemic struck air transport most severely, since a cumulative decline of up to 80% was recorded in Poland in this sector over the entire period of the pandemic.

Another category subject to analysis was individual passenger transport (car sharing, car rental) and taxi services. According to information from the industry, this service sector witnessed a decline of up to 65% (Figure 5.4b) compared to the previous year (Table 5.12 and Figure 5.4a).

Based on the case study, the average share of age groups among passengers and operators participating in various passenger transport services was also determined.

Using the data sets thus compiled, the author determined the total mortality indicators as well as mortality factors broken down into age groups for passenger transport services. The results are summarised in Tables 5.13 and 5.14.

The aggregated total mortality rates established for passenger transport services for the variants and figures assumed are provided in Table 5.15. Car sharing and car rental services have not been included in the collation since they involve participation only of a single passenger (driver) or their family members which entails no random virus transmission.

In order to estimate the number of persons exposed to and the effects (mortality) of the SARS-CoV-2 infection for other freight transport

Table 5.12 Quantitative year-over-year comparison of total passenger transport figures for corresponding periods including the pandemic in Poland

Passenger transport (total) ('000)							
Year	III	IV	V	VI	VII	VIII	IX
2019	54,345	52,298	54,573	50905	43,559	44,070	54,468
2020	32,498	11,455	14,826	21,523	26,458	29,107	37,469
2019	100%	100%	100%	100%	100%	100%	100%
2020	60%	22%	27%	42%	61%	66%	69%

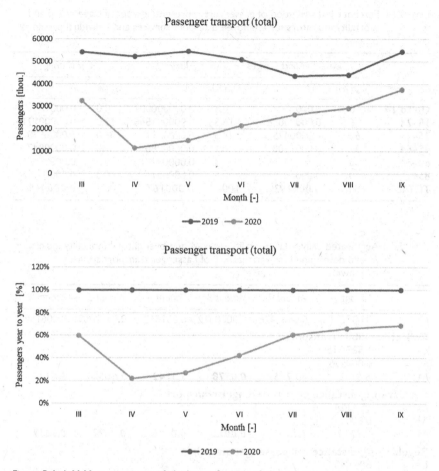

Figure 5.4a,b YoY comparison of declining figures of the passenger transport sector in corresponding periods including the pandemic in Poland.

Table 5.13 Percentage distribution of passengers representing a specific age group and mortality indicators for regular long-distance passenger transport services

Age group (years)	Coach services		Railway		Air transport	
	O_a (%)	M_i	O_a (%)	M_i	O_a (%)	M_i
Up to 14	4.0	0.000000052	5.0	0.000000065	1.1	0.000000014
15–24	44.0	0.000004123	5.0	0.000000469	20.0	0.000001874
25–44	40.0	0.0000274	34.0	0.0000233	50.0	0.0000343
45–64	8.0	0.0000375	46.0	0.0002156	23.0	0.0001079
65–84	4.0	0.000088	8.0	0.000177	5.2	0.000114
85+	0.0	0.000	2.0	0.000203	0.9	0.000091
TOTAL	*100*	**0.000157**	*100*	**0.000619**	*100*	**0.000349**

Table 5.14 Percentage distribution of passengers representing a specific age group and mortality indicators for employee transport services and individual passenger transport

Age group	Employee transport services		Taxi		Car sharing	
	O_a (%)	M_i	O_a (%)	M_i	O_a (%)	M_i
Up to 14	0	0.000	0.5	0.000000007	0.0	0.000
15–24	6	0.000000562	16.5	0.000001546	13.0	0.000001218
25–44	62	0.0000425	74.5	0.0000511	86.0	0.0000590
45–64	32	0.0001500	6.1	0.0000286	1.0	0.0000047
65–84	0	0.000	1.4	0.000031	0.0	0.000
85+	0	0.000	0.5	0.000051	0.0	0.000
TOTAL	100	**0.000193**	100	**0.000163**	100	**0.000065**

Table 5.15 Aggregated daily total mortality rates M_t and overall total mortality indicators M_i and determined for variants 1–6 of passenger transport services nationwide

	Variant 1	Variant 2	Variant 3	Variant 4	Variant 5	Variant 6
I_a	0.0072111	0.0463426	0.0000612	0.0016128	0.0392069	0.0061507
Collective public transport						
L	1,588,315					
M_i	0.000595					
M_t	**6.8148**	**43.7959**	**0.0578**	**1.5242**	**37.0524**	**5.8127**
Regular long-distance coach passenger transport						
L	157,124					
M_i	0.000157					
M_t	**0.1779**	**1.1432**	**0.0015**	**0.0398**	**0.9672**	**0.1517**
Regular long-distance rail passenger transport						
L	597.045					
M_i	0.000619					
M_t	**2.6650**	**17.1269**	**0.0226**	**0.5960**	**14.4897**	**2.2731**
Air passenger transport						
L	11,991					
M_i	0.000349					
M_t	**0.0302**	**0.1939**	**0.0003**	**0.0067**	**0.1641**	**0.0257**
Employee transport services						
L	78,868					
M_i	0.000193					
M_t	**0.1098**	**0.7054**	**0.0009**	**0.0245**	**0.5968**	**0.0936**
Taxi						
L	11,215					
M_i	0.000613					
M_t	**0.0496**	**0.3186**	**0.0004**	**0.0111**	**0.2695**	**0.0423**
ΣM_t	**9.847**	**63.284**	**0.084**	**2.202**	**53.540**	**8.399**

Table 5.15(a) Aggregated daily total mortality rates M_t and overall total mortality indicators M_i and determined for variants 1–6 of underground railway services (as part of collective public transport) nationwide

	Variant 1	Variant 2	Variant 3	Variant 4	Variant 5	Variant 6
I_a	0.0072111	0.0463426	0.0000612	0.0016128	0.0392069	0.0061507
Underground railway						
L	198,740					
M_i	0.000595					
M_t	**0.8527**	**5.4800**	**0.0072**	**0.1907**	**4.6362**	**0.7273**

services, these services were grouped into heavy transport (more than 3.5 tonnes) and individual delivery services, such as catering and grocery deliveries.

Commercial heavy freight services comprise transport of various types of cargo by vehicles with a maximum permissible load capacity of more than 3.5 tonnes. Currently, this market segment is largely dominated by universal transport services using a tractor and semi-trailer combination with a load capacity of 24 tonnes. Based on an analysis of YoY data compilations including periods corresponding to the time of the pandemic (see Figure 5.5), the average decline of the number of transport services provided in this sector was assumed at 12%, hence the forecasted annual mass of cargo shipped by road transport in 2020 which may come to ca. 1,690,544,240 tonnes.

Another freight transport service category is individual transport including direct delivery to the customer. Due to the social situation during the pandemic and various restrictions, food (catering) and grocery (supermarkets) delivery services became very important in this group of services. It is for these services that an increase in the overall figures was recorded against the corresponding period of the previous year, estimated at up to 50%.

Compared to passenger transport, it is significantly more difficult to estimate the number of persons participating in freight transport services who are exposed to viral infection. It is a mistake to assume that epidemic risks can be disregarded for freight transport, especially when considering the droplet route of virus transmission. It is also erroneous to assume that only two persons (driver and customer) are exposed to such a risk. Analogically to the courier parcel delivery services discussed above, the author recommends to analyse the chain of events on the basis of process maps previously prepared for groups of transport services.

Following an analysis of the heavy transport process, the following chain of events involving people was defined: handover of shipment documents – two persons, loading and unloading – four persons, and where drivers participate in the loading and unloading processes, they should also be taken

Table 5.16 Quantitative year-over-year comparison of total road freight transport figures for corresponding periods including the pandemic in Poland

Freight transport (road) ('000 tonnes)

Year	III	IV	V	VI	VII	VIII	IX
2019	24,394	25,225	27,051	26,052	26,099	25,900	24,845
2020	23,753	22,397	22,277	22,609	23,114	21,428	22,928
2019	100%	100%	100%	100%	100%	100%	100%
2020	97%	89%	82%	87%	89%	83%	92%

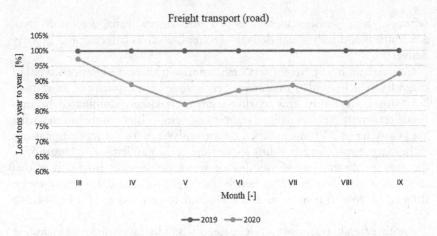

Figure 5.5 Decrease in the amount of cargo shipped by road transport against the corresponding period of the pandemic (year-over-year).

into account in this chain. One can also include the person responsible for securing or preparing the cargo. Consequently, the total number of persons exposed to the epidemic threat and participating in the chain of events for a single heavy transport service may vary between 4 and 6. Hence, the average value of 5 was assumed in the calculations. In order to estimate the average number of transport services performed per day, it was assumed that the total average daily amount of cargo shipped by heavy road transport should be divided by the permissible load capacity of the vehicles used to deliver these transport services, which is 24 tonnes. Hence, the average value of 192,985 vehicles (shipments) daily performing heavy road transport services across the entire country (Poland). Assuming the mean number of five persons involved in the related chain of events for every such transport service, the total daily number of persons exposed to viral infection in the execution of heavy transport processes is 964,923 nationwide.

For direct food or grocery delivery services, the number of persons exposed to viral infection can be estimated by analogy to the courier services involving direct delivery. It is assumed that one driver delivers food to 12 customers per day on average. With regard to direct grocery deliveries, the number of customers averages 30 per day. The chain of events should each time include additional two persons preparing the delivery on site. Having made such assumptions, one can establish the average total number of persons exposed to the risk of viral infection in food delivery services and grocery delivery services at 15 and 33, respectively. What poses a major difficulty in estimating the number of services of this type provided daily is the lack of adequate data. Therefore, a detailed case study was conducted, separately for food and grocery deliveries. Based on statistical data, it was established that the number of catering entities operating in Poland was 20,260, and under normal circumstances home delivery services were offered by about 20% of them, but due to the restrictions imposed on them during the pandemic, the number of home delivery operators increased to 60%, i.e. 12,156. Having made the relevant assumptions linked with the chain of events in question, one can estimate the daily number of persons involved in the food delivery process at 182,340. For home delivery of groceries, hypermarkets, supermarkets and discount stores were taken into consideration. During the pandemic, the number of stores which started offering home deliveries increased significantly (by more than 30%), and so of the 7,000 stores subject to the analysis, ca. 2,100 rendered home delivery services. Assuming that the chain of events involved in grocery deliveries is analogical to that described above, the estimated number of persons participating in the grocery delivery process per day comes to 67,200.

Based on the case study, the average share of age groups among operators and customers participating in various cargo transport services was also determined.

Using the data sets thus compiled, the author determined total mortality indicators as well as mortality factors broken down into age groups for freight transport services. The results are summarised in Table 5.17.

The aggregated total mortality rates established for freight transport services for the variants and figures assumed have been provided in Table 5.18. Rail and air freight transport have been disregarded in this collation, since no door-to-door deliveries are performed in these modes, and they depend on the internal organisation of work by transport operators, which practically excludes direct contact with consumers.

Table 5.17 Percentage distribution of passengers representing a specific age group and mortality indicators for freight transport services

Age group (years)	Heavy transport		Food delivery		Grocery delivery	
	O_a (%)	M_i	O_a (%)	M_i	O_a (%)	M_i
Up to 14	0.0	0.00	0.0	0.00	0.0	0.00
15–24	21.0	0.000001968	40.0	0.000003748	15.0	0.000001406
25–44	76.0	0.0000521	55.0	0.0000377	75.0	0.0000515
45–64	3.0	0.0000141	5.0	0.0000234	10.0	0.0000469
65–84	0.0	0.00	0.0	0.00	0.0	0.00
85+	0.0	0.00	0.0	0.00	0.0	0.00
TOTAL	*100*	**0.000068**	*100*	**0.000065**	*100*	**0.00010**

Table 5.18 Aggregated daily total mortality rates M_t and overall total mortality indicators M_i and determined for variants 1–6 of freight transport services nationwide

	Variant 1	Variant 2	Variant 3	Variant 4	Variant 5	Variant 6
I_a	0.0072111	0.0463426	0.0000612	0.0016128	0.0392069	0.0061507
Courier parcel delivery services						
L	747,640					
M_i	0.000051					
M_t	0.2750	1.7670	0.0023	0.0615	1.4949	0.2345
Heavy transport (above 3.5 tonnes)						
L	964,923					
M_i	0.000068					
M_t	0.4732	3.0408	0.0040	0.1058	2.5726	0.4036
Food delivery						
L	182,340					
M_i	0.000065					
M_t	0.0855	0.5493	0.0007	0.0191	0.4647	0.0729
Grocery delivery						
L	67,200					
M_i	0.00010					
M_t	0.0485	0.3114	0.0004	0.0108	0.2635	0.0413
ΣM_t	**0.8820**	**5.6685**	**0.0075**	**0.1973**	**4.7956**	**0.7523**

5.6 DISCUSSION

Having performed a cumulative analysis of all predefined types of transport services in a breakdown into passenger and freight transport, one can directly compare the relevant services and determine total effects of epidemic threats for the entire transport sector on a nationwide scale.

An additional advantage of the original assumption that the said effects would be estimated for the entire country in a one-day time horizon is that one can take different quantitative share values of specific types of transport services into account, and consequently also consider the scale effect vis-à-vis the nationwide evolution of the epidemic.

Additionally, simulation analyses were performed in order to determine the ratio of deaths estimated as a total mortality rate on account of the coronavirus infection across the sector of transport services to the total number of deaths attributable to COVID-19 over the period analysed (Table 5.19).

However, these results should be regarded as illustrative due to the diverse daily share of transport work (average daily values were assumed in the simulation) and the time shift resulting from different disease duration times, which may span as long as several dozen days from infection to death. In this case, in order to calculate the relevant indicators, one should take the cumulative number of deaths on the given day divided by the cumulative number of cases a certain number of days earlier, where the number of days is the delay taken into account. In a model developed by researchers from the University of Warsaw, delays of 1–7, 10 and 14 days were considered. The maximum fatality rate value thus obtained (for a delay of 14 days) was 5.89%, while the minimum one (for a delay of 0 days) was 4.54%.

The methodology developed by the author makes it possible to analyse the percentage share of estimated fatal effects of COVID-19 attributable to infections associated with diverse transport services. A sample collation of the variants analysed is provided in Table 5.20, expressed in values of proportion to the actual number of deaths.

The values established for variants 5 and 6 should be considered as the most reliable values of the ratio of estimated fatalities due to infection in the transport sector and the daily number of deaths attributable to COVID-19. Variant 5 corresponds to the values averaged for the worst month in terms

Table 5.19 Comparison of the number of deaths due to COVID-19 with the estimated total mortality rate attributable to the SARS-CoV-2 infection in the transport sector in Poland for variants 1–6 subject to analysis

	Variant 1	Variant 2	Variant 3	Variant 4	Variant 5	Variant 6
A **Deaths due to COVID-19**	45.8889	674	1.1786	10.2581	378.9000	63.0515
B ΣM_t	10.7293	68.9524	0.0911	2.3997	58.3353	9.1515
B/A [%]	23.38%	10.23%	7.73%	23.39%	15.40%	14.51%

Table 5.20 Percentage share of estimated fatalities due to COVID-19 attributable to infections associated with different transport services against the actual number of fatalities

	Variant 1	Variant 2	Variant 3	Variant 4	Variant 5	Variant 6
Actual fatalities	45.89	674	1.18	10.26	378.90	63.05
Courier services	0.60%	0.26%	0.20%	0.60%	0.39%	0.37%
Heavy transport	1.03%	0.45%	0.34%	1.03%	0.68%	0.64%
Food delivery	0.19%	0.08%	0.06%	0.19%	0.12%	0.12%
Grocery delivery	0.11%	0.05%	0.03%	0.11%	0.07%	0.07%
Public transport	14.85%	6.50%	4.91%	14.86%	9.78%	9.22%
Regular coach	0.39%	0.17%	0.13%	0.39%	0.26%	0.24%
Long-distance railway	5.81%	2.54%	1.92%	5.81%	3.82%	3.61%
Air transport	0.07%	0.03%	0.02%	0.07%	0.04%	0.04%
Employee transport	0.24%	0.10%	0.08%	0.24%	0.16%	0.15%
Taxi	0.11%	0.05%	0.04%	0.11%	0.07%	0.07%
Total	23.38%	10.23%	7.73%	23.39%	15.40%	14.51%

of the epidemic status in Poland (with the highest number of active cases and fatalities). Variant 6 represents the overall evolution of the coronavirus pandemic in Poland to date. Although the percentage values established for these two variants differ to a slight extent, as the standard deviation is 0.445 (0.89%), however, compared to the other values provided in Table 5.19 and depending on the choice of the test sample and period, the differences can be considerable, scattered over the range of more than 15%. A graphical comparison of the said two variants is provided in Figure 5.6.

To verify the models developed by the author, they were compared with real-life data spanning 8 months of the epidemic evolution in Poland. The results thus obtained have been provided in the diagram below. The graph features an additional curve representing active COVID-19 cases, since the model is linked with the daily indicator of active SARS-CoV-2 infection cases (I_a) (Figure 5.7).

5.7 CONCLUSIONS

Given the universal and common nature of transport as it functions in the country's public and economic domain, it was assumed that the effects of epidemic threats should be analysed on a nationwide scale. The epidemic situation which constitutes the subject matter of this monograph is associated with the SARS-CoV-2 coronavirus epidemic, which has evolved into a global pandemic. Therefore, limiting the analysis of such effects to

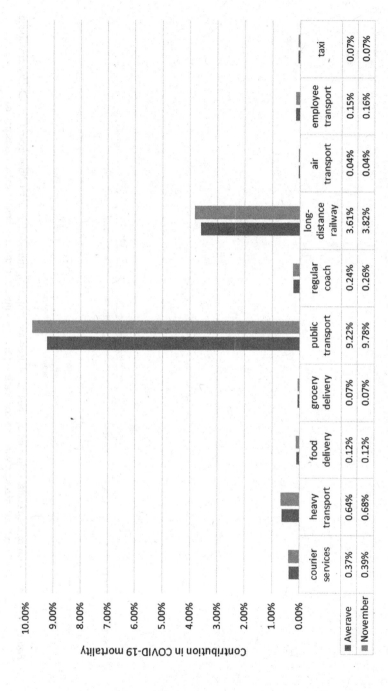

Figure 5.6 Percentage share of estimated fatalities due to COVID-19 attributable to infections associated with different transport services compared to the actual number of fatalities.

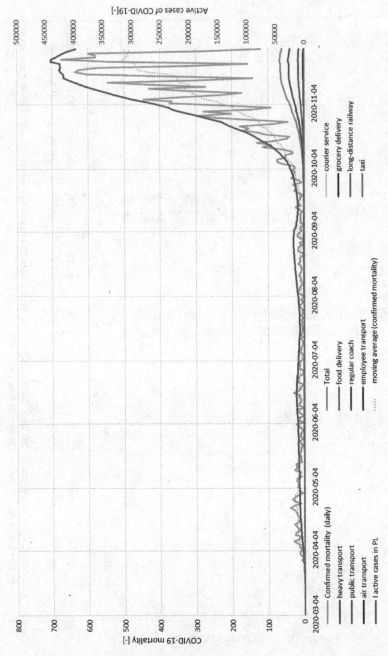

Figure 5.7 Comparison of the results delivered by the model used for estimating the number of fatalities from COVID-19 attributable to transport-related infection with the confirmed mortality values and the number of active cases per day.

a single instance of a transport service delivery seems illegitimate, as the consequences in question affect the entire society. However, the methodology developed by the author for the purpose of estimating the effects of epidemic threats attributable to transport services is universal. Based on complete disclosure and mathematic formalisation, this method is suitable for application against any chosen criteria. It can be expanded or limited geographically, from the scale of a single municipality to that of the entire world. It can be narrowed down to a specific company or even a single service provision case. All depends on the assumed goal of the analysis and the available data. The estimation ranges obviously also depend on the nature of the epidemic threat.

What this method uses is a set of statistical indicators, but each of them has been defined mathematically which makes it possible to establish the values of these indicators each time depending on the area of application of the method in question (e.g. another country, worldwide, specific business, etc.). Moreover, this method can be applied to any other epidemic, yet this would require compilation of a similar set of data characterising the given epidemic and appropriate adjustment of the values of the relevant indicators, including activity and mortality.

The author has also proposed an interesting data estimation solution, which proves particularly helpful in the absence of detailed real-life data on the transport sector, based on case studies, process maps and chains of events.

All of the foregoing proves a great application potential of the method addressed in this monograph.

The methodology proposed for estimation of the effects of viral infection attributable to transport services can significantly complement the methodology of the epidemic evolution studies and represent an important source of knowledge to be used when identifying process-related (non-stationary) epidemic outbreaks. It should also be taken into consideration in epidemic evolution forecasting models correlated with relevant transport sector projections. Owing to the open nature of the methodology, it can also function as a very important source of knowledge enabling identification of infection mechanisms, and consequently prove particularly useful when developing dedicated spot epidemic control strategies.

Chapter 6

Comprehensive Method of Epidemic Risk Assessment in Transport

6.1 PRINCIPLES OF THE COMPREHENSIVE METHOD OF EPIDEMIC RISK ASSESSMENT IN TRANSPORT

If, according to the most general definition, the probability of an adverse event taking place is assumed as the risk, then the values established in line with the methodology discussed in Chapter 4 will be the measures of the risk of viral infection in transport services. What applies in this case is the definition of the risk score designed to represent an underlying probability of an adverse event denoted as Y given a vector of P explaining variables X containing measurements of the relevant risk factors.

However, in the methodological area of risk management, it is common to distinguish between concepts pertaining only to the probability of an adverse event taking place and the broader concept of risk, which is additionally analysed against the effects of the adverse event and sometimes also assigned a measure of exposure to that event. A sphere in which risk assessment is considered particularly important, and consequently also where one can find the most risk assessment methods and measures, is that of ergonomics and occupational safety. With regard to workplaces, occupational risk assessment methods refer to these effects by considering accident rates or costs, while exposure is addressed from the perspective of exposure time or measures of substance concentration. For the epidemic risk assessment performed in transport, some other risk assessment criteria should be proposed.

This becomes even more relevant in light of the current research. Based on air travel data, studies assessed the risk of potential international spread of the disease at early stages (Lai et al., 2020; Bogoch et al., 2020). Additionally, significant correlations were found between case numbers and the volume of domestic transport, including flights, trains and buses (Zheng, R et al., 2020). Travel restrictions and social distancing measures have been introduced across countries to contain or mitigate the SARS-CoV-2 transmission. However, only meta-population-level transport data and models

DOI: 10.1201/9781003204732-6

were used in those studies to measure the potential risk of seeding the virus between locations (Kucharski et al., 2020; Hellewell et al., 2020), and yet it remains unknown how coronavirus transmits between individual travellers using specific transport modes (Hu et al., 2020).

One should also mind the subject-oriented nature of risk assessment, the subject being the risk target. Risk and its assessment criteria should be defined differently when assessing threats to an individual person. If the risk is analysed in a general context, for example, that of a business, an industry, a country or, as in this case, the development of an epidemic, the assessment should be based on different criteria and scales.

With regard to risk assessment, one must follow the procedure of scale determination and scoring. Risk scoring is the process of attaining a calculated score that provides information on how severe a risk is based on several factors. It is very important to select a scoring system to help identify the most serious hazards. That is precisely why there are many risk assessment methods dedicated to specific applications (industries). The author has decided to propose a risk assessment method dedicated to the transport sector and implemented in light of epidemic threats.

6.2 MULTI-CRITERIA METHOD FOR TRANSPORT-ASSOCIATED EPIDEMIC RISK ASSESSMENT

What ensures that a risk assessment matches its actual effects is a set of correctly defined impact factors and corresponding partial rating scales. The author typically claims that each and every objective quantitative assessment is only as good as its partial scales, making it possible to assign correct values of the quantitative assessment components. When using scales expressed as subjective impressions, representing categories such as *a little – moderately – a lot*, the final assessment, which assumes the form of a value, can hardly be perceived as an objective quantitative measure because it is developed on the grounds of subjective partial measures. That is why it is particularly important to develop measurable partial assessment scales in a thorough manner.

With regard to the problem subject to analysis, i.e. assessment of the risk of viral infection in transport, which is very important for the dynamics of epidemic transmission and for implementation of adequate and effective restrictions in the area of transport at a national (regional) scale, the following impact factors were identified for purposes of the risk level assessment:

- probability of infection (viral pathogen transmission) attributable to a transport service (at a single service scale),
- exposure – mean time of direct contact between participants in a transport process (at a single service scale),

- effects – case fatality rate (total mortality rate) for a specific group of transport services as the potential total number of persons who have died due to being infected with the SARS-CoV-2 virus while participating in a transport process (at a daily scale nationwide),
- number of exposed persons – number of persons involved in a chain of events within a certain unit of time of process implementation (at a single service scale).

The multiplicative coefficient of R_{eT} was assumed as the measure of the epidemic risk assessment for transport, given by the following formula:

$$R_{eT} = P_i \cdot E_i \cdot M_{ti} \cdot L_i \tag{6.1}$$

where:

P_i – probability of infection (viral pathogen transmission) attributable to the ith transport service (Table 4.19),

E_i – exposure time, i.e. mean time of direct contact between participants of the ith transport process,

M_{ti} – total mortality rate of a specific group of transport services, understood as the potential total number of persons who have died due to being infected with the SARS-CoV-2 virus while participating in the ith transport process at a daily scale nationwide (Tables 5.15 and 5.18),

L_i – number of exposed persons, i.e. the number of persons involved in a chain of events within a certain unit of time of process implementation (30 min).

The transport-associated infection probability factor is inextricably linked with the criterion of the adverse event occurrence risk, which makes it a strong determinant of the overall risk assessment. The methodology for estimating this probability, as extensively discussed in Chapter 4, is based on a premise that the final measure is calculated for a single transport service provision on the basis of process maps by taking all potential virus transmission mechanisms into account.

The assumed measure of exposure is the mean time of direct contact between the participants in the transport process, and its relevance for the probability of droplet viral infection is dominant, and also, which is particularly worth noting, it increases the probability of contact virus transmission on account of the increased frequency of contact with surfaces or skin on which the pathogen may potentially persist.

Another risk assessment factor is that of infection effects. On account of the lack of access to a complete database of effects of the SARS-CoV-2 virus infection or COVID-19, as well as the complete inability to link the effects to the infections attributable to transport services, it was the estimated number of fatalities due to COVID-19 which the author adopted as a measure of the effects. The entire methodology for estimating the effects of viral infection in transport services by taking into consideration the mortality rates established on the basis of the distribution of predefined age groups has been discussed in Chapter 5. In this case, given the assumption that the risk assessment should pertain to the nationwide scale of the epidemic evolution and the diversified impact of different shares of transport services on it, the measure in question was analysed against daily rates for the entire country.

The last factor included in the multi-criteria method for transport-associated epidemic risk assessment is the number of persons exposed to an adverse event. This is an extremely important assessment criterion because it largely determines the values in most epidemic models as the number of infected persons who are potential virus carriers. They are the ones responsible for subsequent infections as well as for the geographical spread of the epidemic. Using the methodology developed by the author, one could determine this number by analysing the chain of contact events, as described in Chapter 5. Given the current state of knowledge about the notion of virus infectivity, this value is established as the number of persons involved in the chain of events within a specific unit of time of the process implementation at a scale of a single service. On account of the probability of droplet infection, the time unit assumed for the sake of population count was 30 min. For services where the entire process involves participation of a fixed number of persons (e.g. passengers) for more than 30 min, for example, air transport, this value was calculated once and had a constant value. Where the provision of a single service may be shorter, for example, in underground railway transport, the final value should be adjusted against the 30-min unit by taking the number of vehicle filling operations into consideration (e.g. 2.5) since there is an exchange of passengers within the analysed interval of 30 min. When estimating this figure for freight transport, the only contacts whose time is to be accounted for are those between the driver and the customer, or between the driver and the warehouseman, etc.

In order to determine the final assessment score based on the partial scores obtained for the aforementioned factors, also the factors of impact on the final epidemic risk should be analysed. It would be incorrect to assume that each of these factors determines the final risk score to the same extent. Therefore, in order to develop rating scales for these factors by considering how they affect the final risk, an analytic hierarchy process (AHP), described more extensively in Chapter 3, was performed in order to establish the significance levels and weights of individual factors towards the risk of infection in transport. The results thus obtained are provided in Table 6.1.

Table 6.1 Results of the AHP and weighting factors for transport-associated infection risk assessment factors

Pairwise comparison matrix A\B	Transmission probability	Exposure (transport time)	Mortality rate	Number of infected persons	AHP weighting factor
Infection probability	1	2	5	1/2	**0.30**
Exposure (transport time)	1/2	1	3	1/3	**0.17**
Mortality rate	1/5	1/3	1	1/5	**0.07**
Number of infected persons	2	3	5	1	**0.47**

The matrix thus obtained is consistent since its maximum eigenvalue is λ_{max}=4.055, while its consistency index (CI)=0.0183 and its consistency ratio (CR)=0.0204, which is a satisfactory value, being much smaller than 0.1. Consequently, the weighting factors thus calculated constituted the starting point for developing dedicated scales for the assessment of partial factors.

One should also note the assumptions made and the interpretation in the hierarchical assessment. The significance of the relevant factors of probability, exposure, effect and number of exposed persons were analysed against the factors determining the dynamics of the epidemic changes based on the models deployed, as described in Chapters 4 and 5 of the monograph. Additionally, the epidemic status of the entire country was assumed as the analytical scale – hence such a high hierarchical assessment of the number of exposed persons, since it is these persons who may become subsequent individuals spreading the infection, which is the most important factor in epidemic models (SIR and SEIR). Pathogen transmission probability was addressed next as the quantity which determines the number of successful virus transmissions. The relevance of exposure time is predominant in this respect, but only in a single-case analysis, which is why its importance dwindles when the assessment is performed at a global scale. The risk effects, defined as the mortality rate (number of deaths), no longer have a direct impact on further virus transmission, but are by far the most important social and civilisational effects, which is precisely why they were taken into account under the risk assessment.

Based on the weighting factors computed, determining the level of significance of the partial factors assumed in the risk assessment, specific scale ranges were proposed. Following the principle of proportionality, the following upper thresholds of the scoring scales were adopted:

- for the number of exposed persons – maximum value of 50 (weighting factor of 0.47),

- for transmission probability – maximum value of 30 (weighting factor of 0.30),
- for exposure time – maximum value of 15 (weighting factor of 0.17),
- for effects (daily mortality rate in Poland) – maximum value of 10 (weighting coefficient of 0.07).

The next step consisted in establishing the elementary ranges which should be adequate to the function representing the relevant phenomena, i.e. characterise the distribution of the values of the partial factors across the entire transport sector with reference to representative transport services. A decided majority of the characteristics of these phenomena have been described and analysed in previous chapters. However, some hierarchical aggregate functions were additionally established for consecutive partial risk assessment factors (Figures 6.1–6.4).

Based on the established approximation functions, representing distributions of the values obtained for the criteria analysed across the entire sector of transport services (i.e. both passenger and freight transport), and taking into account the weighting factors representing the level of significance of the given factor used in the assessment of the transport-associated epidemic risk, dedicated scales were developed for the factors subject to analysis, as provided in Table 6.2.

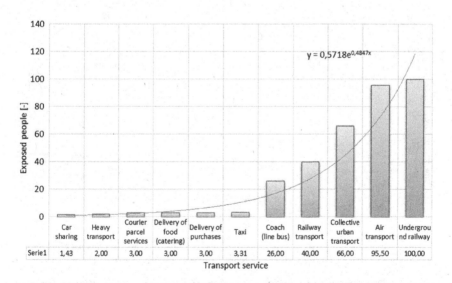

Figure 6.1 Distribution and function of the number of persons exposed to viral infection for individual groups of transport services (30-min interval).

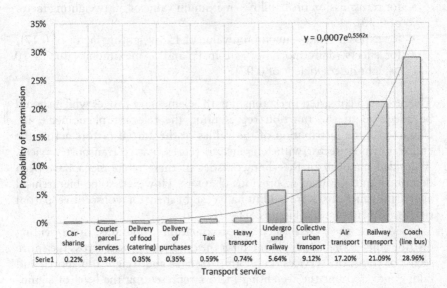

Figure 6.2 Distribution and function of the probability of viral pathogen transmission for individual groups of transport services (30-min interval).

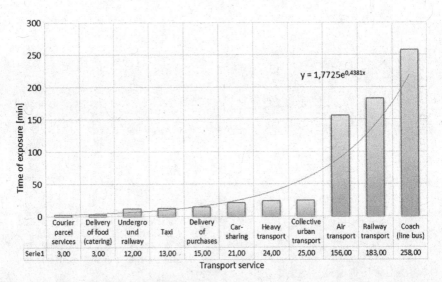

Figure 6.3 Distribution and function of the time of exposure to viral infection for individual groups of transport services (30-min interval).

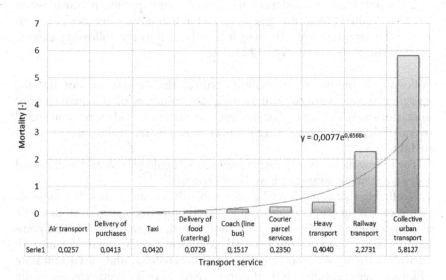

Figure 6.4 Distribution and function of the effects (number of fatalities) attributable to potential viral infection for individual groups of transport services (per day, nationwide).

Table 6.2 Scales defined for the assessment of the transport-associated viral infection risk factors

Score	No. of exposed persons	Score	Transmission probability [%]	Score	Exposure time	Score	Mortality
0,1	[0–1]	0,5	[0–0.25]	0,1	[0–5]	1	[0–0.05]
0,5	(1–2]	1	(0.25–0.5]	0,5	(5–10]	2	(0.05–0.1]
5	(2–5]	3	(0.5–1]	1	(10–15]	3	(0.1–0.2]
10	(5–15]	5	(1–3]	2	(15–20]	4	(0.2–0.3]
15	(15–30]	7	(3–5]	3	(20–25]	5	(0.3–0.4]
20	(30–45]	10	(5–8]	5	(25–30]	6	(0.4–0.5]
30	(45–60]	15	(8–12]	7	(30–60]	7	(0.5–1]
35	(60–75]	20	(12–20]	10	(60–90]	8	(1–5]
40	(75–90]	25	(20–30]	12	(90–120]	9	(5–10]
50	>90	30	>30	15	>120	10	>10

The possible values of R_{eT} ranged between 0.005 and 225,000. And consecutively, for the following cases:

1   number of exposed persons within the range of 0–1, viral pathogen transmission up to 0.25%, exposure time up to 5 min and daily number of potential fatalities up to 0.05, which translates into the following expression: $R_{eT} = 0.1 \cdot 0.5 \cdot 0.1 \cdot 1 = 0.005$;

2   number of exposed persons over 90, viral pathogen transmission over 30%, exposure time over 120 min and daily number of potential fatalities over 10, which translates into the following expression: $R_{eT} = 50 \cdot 30 \cdot 15 \cdot 10 = 225,000$.

Following a multi-variant analysis, critical threshold values of the R_{eT} epidemic threat factor as well as adequate strategies of risk management operations were identified. The risk level classifications and the recommended overall risk management strategies, as proposed by the author, are described in Table 6.3.

The following levels of transport-associated epidemic risk and operational risk management strategies have been proposed.

Negligible risk which may be acceptable. What the author recommends in this case is an observation strategy based on periodical control measures and environment monitoring. This implies both internal (specific to a company or service sector) and external monitoring of the environment with particular attention to the development of the epidemic and the current state of knowledge regarding viral infection. Based on past experience, especially related to the consequences of the SARS-CoV-2 pandemic, it is reasonable to assume that such an approach in transport-associated risk management should already function as the starting point and have been implemented for good in the transport sector.

The next level comprises low risk. Where the value of R_{eT} ranges between 101 and 15,000, a preparation for change strategy should be applied. It is based on threat identification and assessment, for instance, by the DHI

Table 6.3 R_{eT} scale of transport-associated epidemic risk assessment and matching operational strategies

R_{eT}	Risk level	Strategy
0.005–100	Negligible / acceptable	Observation strategy based on periodical control measures and environment monitoring
101–15,000	Low	Strategy of preparation for change based on identification and assessment of threat, ongoing monitoring of risk factors, as well as environment adaptation to the changes (technical support)
15,001– 30,000	Significant	Strategy of changes based on successive implementation of corrective measures intended to minimise the risk at hand (procedures and technical support)
30,001– 60,000	High	Strategy of instantaneous changes based on actions that eliminate risk factors or reduce its effects (restrictions)
> 60,000	Very high / unacceptable	Containment strategy based on measures that temporarily ban the provision of services or on introduction of alternative services

method described in Chapter 3, as well as continuous monitoring of risk factors. The actions undertaken as a part of this strategy should also include adaptation of the environment (including the supra level and the transport infrastructure) to the changes observed in order to minimise the epidemic risk factors (through projects, concepts and analyses). Some examples of the foregoing may be concepts for technical systems of support for epidemic safety in transport and general organisational recommendations for different operational scenarios.

Another level of epidemic risk has been designated as significant. The change strategies recommended in this case are based on successive implementation of corrective measures aimed at risk minimisation. These measures should be systemic in terms of the technical support for epidemic safety in transport as well as the dedicated procedures and recommendations which are adequate to the current epidemic situation. If the risk level has evolved from negligible to significant, at this stage, one should use the findings from the analyses and concepts conceived in the previous level (low).

Where the risk is classified as high ($30,001 < R_{eT} < 60,000$), the recommendations of the instantaneous change strategy should be deployed at once. This requires measures aimed at eliminating the dominant risk factors or mitigating their effects. It often requires some additional restrictions to be imposed on the provision of services or even on the operation of the entire transport sector.

The last level in the risk classification is very high, which is completely unacceptable. Where this is the case, it is advisable to apply a containment strategy assuming measures that temporarily ban the provision of services or introducing alternative services.

The comprehensive model of epidemic risk management in transport assumes evolutionary development of risks, which allows for specific strategies to be prepared on the grounds of internal actions whenever the epidemic threats resulting from the overall situation increase. Moreover, implementing strategies dedicated to specific risk levels makes it possible to reduce the risk attributable to internal actions, provided that the external epidemic situation remains stable. Consequently, it is possible to seamlessly switch to less restrictive strategies, appropriate for lower risk levels.

6.3 EXAMPLES OF APPLICATION OF THE MULTI-CRITERIA EPIDEMIC RISK ASSESSMENT METHOD IN TRANSPORT FOR REPRESENTATIVE GROUPS OF SERVICES

In line with the methodology developed by the author for the epidemic risk assessment in respect of transport, some representative groups of transport services were analysed. Their synthetic overview has been provided in this chapter.

For the car sharing service, the following partial factor values were calculated:

- average total pathogen transmission probability of 0.22%, as determined with reference to data in Table 4.19,
- average exposure time of 21 min, as determined with reference to the relevant data extracted from a car sharing application,
- factor of effects, understood as the mortality attributable to infection, assumed to be identical as for taxi services, i.e. 0.0423 (Table 5.15), although one could actually adopt the value of zero on account of the absence of droplet infection,
- number of persons exposed obtained by dividing the pre-assumed time unit of 30 min by the exposure time for one driver, i.e. 30/21 = 1.43.

Having assigned the scores according to Table 6.2, one obtains the following:

$$R_{eT} = 0.5 \cdot 3 \cdot 1 \cdot 0.5 = 0.75$$

With regard to the taxi service, the following partial factors were established:

- average total pathogen transmission probability of 0.59%, as determined with reference to data in Table 4.19,
- average exposure time of 13 min, as determined with reference to relevant data obtained from taxi corporations,
- factor of effects, understood as mortality attributable to infection, determined with reference to data in Table 5.15, that is, 0.0423,
- number of persons exposed obtained by dividing the pre-assumed time unit of 30 min by the exposure time for one driver, i.e. 30/13 + 1 = 3.31.

Having assigned the scores according to Table 6.2, one obtains the following:

$$R_{eT} = 3 \cdot 1 \cdot 1 \cdot 5 = 15$$

The following values of partial factors were determined for underground railway:

- average total pathogen transmission probability of 5.64%, as determined with reference to data in Table 4.19,
- average exposure time of 12 min, as determined with reference to the relevant data concerning the Warsaw Metro (underground railway),

- factor of effects, understood as mortality attributable to infection in underground railway, of 0.7273 (Table 5.15(a)),
- number of persons exposed obtained by dividing the pre-assumed time unit of 30 min by the exposure time for a underground railway wagon filled to a half with approximately 121 passengers, i.e. $30/12 \cdot 121.17 = 302.92$.

Having assigned the scores according to Table 6.2, one obtains the following:

$$R_{eT} = 10 \cdot 1 \cdot 7 \cdot 50 = 3500$$

In the case of collective public transport, the following values of partial factors were established:

- average total pathogen transmission probability of 9.12%, as determined with reference to data in Table 4.19,
- average exposure time of 25 min, as determined with reference to the relevant data from comprehensive traffic surveys,
- factor of effects, understood as mortality attributable to infection, of 5.8127, as determined with reference to data in Table 5.15,
- number of persons exposed obtained by dividing the pre-assumed time unit of 30 min by the exposure time for a bus filled to a half with approximately 55 passengers, i.e. $30/25 \cdot 55 = 66$.

Having assigned the scores according to Table 6.2, one obtains the following:

$$R_{eT} = 15 \cdot 3 \cdot 9 \cdot 35 = 14175$$

The following values of partial factors were computed for air passenger transport:

- average total pathogen transmission probability of 17.20%, as determined with reference to data in Table 4.19,
- average exposure time of 156 min, as determined on the basis of the following comparison of selected flights (see Table 6.4),
- factor of effects, understood as mortality attributable to infection, of 0.0257, as determined with reference to data in Table 5.15,
- number of persons exposed due to the travel time without additional passenger flow, assuming half the capacity of a Boeing 737–800 aircraft including the crew, i.e. $191/2 = 95.5$.

Table 6.4 Time of selected popular international flights from Poland

Departure	Arrival	Time (min)
Warszawa, Katowice, Gdańsk, Poznań	Corfu, Greece	150
Warszawa, Katowice, Gdańsk, Poznań, Wrocław, Kraków, Łódź, Bydgoszcz	Crete, Greece	150
Warszawa, Katowice, Gdańsk, Wrocław, Kraków, Bydgoszcz, Rzeszów, Łódź	Kos, Greece	180
Warszawa, Katowice, Gdańsk, Wrocław, Poznań	Tenerife, Spain	300
Warszawa, Łódź, Gdańsk, Katowice, Wrocław, Kraków, Rzeszów, Bydgoszcz	Antalya, Turkey	210
Warszawa, Gdańsk, Wrocław, Kraków, Katowice	Bari, Italy	135
Warszawa, Katowice	London, UK	155
Warszawa	Frankfurt, Germany	125
Warszawa	Oslo, Norway	130
Warszawa	Stockholm, Sweden	110
Warszawa	Dublin, Ireland	180
Warszawa	Brussels, Belgium	130
Warszawa	Amsterdam, The Netherlands	140
Warszawa	Copenhagen, Denmark	95
Average:		**156.43**

Having assigned the scores according to Table 6.2, one obtains the following:

$$R_{eT} = 20 \cdot 15 \cdot 1 \cdot 50 = 15000$$

The following values of partial factors were established for long-distance rail transport:

- average total pathogen transmission probability of 21.09%, as determined with reference to data in Table 4.19,
- average exposure time of 183 min, as determined with reference to the most popular railway services in Poland (see Table 6.5),
- factor of effects, understood as mortality attributable to infection, of 2.2731, as determined with reference to data in Table 5.15,
- number of persons exposed due to the travel time without additional passenger flow, assuming half the capacity of a single passenger train car, i.e. 80/2 = 40.

Having assigned the scores according to Table 6.2, one obtains the following:

Table 6.5 Travel times of selected popular train services in Poland

Departure	Arrival	Time (min)
Warszawa	Gdansk	178
Warszawa	Częstochowa	130
Warszawa	Kraków	150
Warszawa	Katowice	150
Warszawa	Opole	182
Warszawa	Wrocław	220
Warszawa	Poznań	150
Gdansk	Kraków	330
Kraków	Wrocław	190
Katowice	Wrocław	145
Average:		**182.5**

$$R_{eT} = 25 \cdot 15 \cdot 8 \cdot 20 = 60000$$

For national coach bus transport services, the following partial factor values were calculated:

- average total pathogen transmission probability (viral pathogen transmission) of 28.96%, as determined with reference to data in Table 4.19,
- average exposure time of 258 min, as determined with reference to the most popular coach services in Poland (see Table 6.6),
- factor of effects, understood as mortality attributable to infection, of 0.1517, as determined with reference to data in Table 5.15,
- number of persons exposed due to the travel time without additional passenger flow, assuming a half of the seats taken in popular regular coach services, i.e. 50/2+1 = 26.

Having assigned the scores according to Table 6.2, one obtains the following:

$$R_{eT} = 25 \cdot 15 \cdot 3 \cdot 15 = 16875$$

The epidemic risk assessment for freight transport was conducted in an analogical manner by referring to representative groups of transport services. The main difference in terms of the factor analysis lies in the estimation of the number of exposed persons and the exposure time. For freight transport, one should only consider the time of contacts in the driver–customer, driver–warehouseman and similar configurations. In line with such an approach, the number of persons exposed to infection should also be determined with regard to a 30-min interval.

Table 6.6 Travel times of selected popular coach bus services in Poland

Departure	Arrival	Time (min)
Warszawa	Wrocław	260
Wrocław	Łódź	175
Częstochowa	Kraków	125
Gdansk	Poznań	265
Gliwice	Zakopane	285
Katowice	Rzeszów	210
Lublin	Sopot	506
Bełchatów	Wrocław	240
Average:		**258.25**

The first group of analysed freight transport services is courier parcel delivery. The following values of partial factors were determined for this service:

- average total pathogen transmission probability of 0.34%, as determined with reference to data in Table 4.19,
- average exposure time of 3.65 min, as determined on the basis of service time reports for courier–addressee or customer service staff–addressee contacts. This value comprises an averaged time of contact between the warehouseman and the courier, computed per a single delivery service, at the parcel release for shipment;
- factor of effects, understood as mortality attributable to infection, of 0.2345, as determined with reference to data in Table 5.18,
- number of persons exposed resulting from the assumption that within the pre-assumed time unit of 30 min the courier delivers a parcel every 15 min to two addressees on average, hence 30/15 +1 = 3.

Having assigned the scores according to Table 6.2, one obtains the following:

$$R_{eT} = 1 \cdot 0.1 \cdot 4 \cdot 5 = 2$$

Another group of freight transport services taken into consideration is food (catering) delivery. The following values of partial factors were determined for this service:

- average total pathogen transmission probability of 0.35%, as determined with reference to the data in Table 4.19,
- average exposure time of 2.83 min, as determined on the basis of service time reports for courier–customer contacts. This value also

comprises an averaged time of contact between the restaurant worker and the courier, computed per à single delivery service, at the meal handover for delivery;
- factor of effects, understood as mortality attributable to infection, of 0.0729, as determined with reference to data in Table 5.18,
- number of persons exposed resulting from the assumption that within the pre-assumed time unit of 30 min the courier delivers food every 15 min to two customers on average, hence 30/15 +1 = 3.

Having assigned the scores according to Table 6.2, one obtains the following:

$$R_{eT} = 1 \cdot 0.1 \cdot 2 \cdot 5 = 1$$

Also grocery delivery service was analysed as representative of the freight transport sector. The following values of partial factors were determined for this service:

- average total pathogen transmission probability of 0.35%, as determined with reference to data in Table 4.19,
- average exposure time of 16.67 min, as determined on the basis of service time reports for courier–customer contacts. This value also comprises an averaged time assumed to account for the shipment completion and loading at the store, computed per a single delivery service, and the related contact between the store employee and the courier, which approximates to 15 min;
- factor of effects, understood as mortality attributable to infection, of 0.0413, as determined with reference to data in Table 5.18,
- number of persons exposed resulting from the assumption that within the pre-assumed time unit of 30 min the courier delivers groceries every 15 min to two customers on average, hence 30/15 +1 = 3.

Having assigned the scores according to Table 6.2, one obtains the following:

$$R_{eT} = 1 \cdot 2 \cdot 1 \cdot 5 = 10$$

The last group of freight transport services subject to analysis is heavy transport above 3.5 tonnes. The following values of partial factors were determined for this service:

- average total pathogen transmission probability of 0.74%, as determined with reference to data in Table 4.19,

- average exposure time of 24 min, as determined on the basis of service time reports for courier–customer contacts, during which the driver participates in loading or unloading operations. This value comprises averaged time, computed per a single delivery, assuming four destination points per a single service run as well as the times corresponding to the documentation and cargo handover to and verification by the customer at the delivery destination,
- factor of effects, understood as mortality attributable to infection, of 0.4036, as determined with reference to data in Table 5.18,
- number of persons exposed resulting from the assumption that within the pre-assumed time unit of 30 min the driver delivers the cargo to a single customer, hence the value of 2 (driver + customer).

Having assigned the scores according to Table 6.2, one obtains the following:

$$R_{eT} = 3 \cdot 3 \cdot 6 \cdot 0.5 = 27$$

Following the procedure described above, the epidemic risk scores were established for the chosen groups of transport services representative of the entire transport sector.

6.4 DISCUSSION

To compare the epidemic risk established for different groups of transport services, the results previously obtained are summarised in Table 6.7. It provides a comparison of the R_{eT} values calculated for the analysed transport services for mean values of total pathogen transmission probability and assuming the current social distancing restrictions imposed on the transport sector, namely, the obligation to ensure that means of transport are filled up to 50% of their capacity. Averaged values of mortality established for the given group of transport services, calculated for a period since the beginning of the SARS-CoV-2 virus epidemic in Poland, were assumed as the effects included in the risk assessment.

Records in the R_{eT} column have been marked with greyscales that indicate the risk assessment level according to Table 6.3. The epidemic threat was identified as a negligible risk in the case of all freight transport services as well as car sharing and taxi services. A low level risk was assigned to passenger transport by underground railway, collective public transport and air transport. It was estimated that long-distance regular coach services represented a significant risk, while the risk of a high level was identified in long-distance rail transport services.

Table 6.7 Summary of the analysis results and the R_{eT} values obtained from the transport-associated epidemic risk assessment, assuming the applicable restrictions and averaged epidemic rates

Epidemic risk in transport	Score	No. of exposed persons	Score	Transmission probability (%)	Score	Exposure time	Score	Mortality	R_{eT}
Passenger transport									
Car sharing	0.5	1.43	0.5	0.22	3	21.00	1	0.0000	0.75
Taxi	5	3.31	3	0.59	1	13.00	1	0.0423	15
Underground railway	50	302.92	10	5.64	1	12.00	7	0.7273	3,500
Collective urban transport	35	66.00	15	9.12	3	25.00	9	5.8127	14,175
Air transport	50	95.50	20	17.20	15	156.00	1	0.0257	15,000
Railway transport	20	40.00	25	21.09	15	183.00	8	2.2731	60,000
Regular coach services	15	26.00	25	28.96	15	258.00	3	0.1517	16,875
Freight transport									
Courier parcel delivery services	5	3.00	1	0.34	0.1	3.65	4	0.2345	2
Food delivery (catering)	5	3.00	1	0.35	0.1	2.83	2	0.0729	1
Grocery delivery	5	3.00	1	0.35	2	16.67	1	0.0413	10
Heavy transport	0.5	2.00	3	0.74	3	24.00	6	0.4036	27

The above transport-associated epidemic risk assessments based on the R_{eT} coefficient apply to the assumptions described in Chapters 4 and 5 for variant 6, which includes components of average values determined over the long-term period of analysis of the SARS-CoV-2 virus epidemic in Poland, i.e. from March to November 2020. However, following an analysis of the differences in the statistical values concerning the effects, i.e. the estimated number of fatalities attributable to viral infection in transport, for the six variants analysed (Chapter 5), and additionally taking into account the significant differences in the values of the viral pathogen transmission probability depending on the chosen variant of the transport service provision process, as presented in Chapter 4, one should note that there are considerable differences between individual final epidemic risk assessments depending on the scenarios referred to in terms of the overall epidemic situation and the service delivery variant.

Therefore, for the sake of comparison, the epidemic risk assessment values have been compared against a case of no restrictions imposed in terms of wearing protective masks and social distancing, i.e. assuming that the full capacity of the relevant means of transport is used. Also for this case, the assessment of effects was assumed to be based on the estimated mortality rate on the worst day of the epidemic in Poland in terms of the number of fatalities attributable to COVID-19 (25 November 2020, variant 2) (Table 6.8).

Table 6.8 Summary of the analysis results and the R_{eT} values obtained from the transport-associated epidemic risk assessment, assuming no restrictions and the worst epidemic rates

Epidemic risk in transport	Score	No. of exposed persons	Score	Transmission probability (%)	Score	Exposure time	Score	Mortality	R_{eT}
Passenger transport									
Car sharing	0.5	1.43	0.5	0.22	3	21.00	1	0.0000	0.75
Taxi	5	3.31	5	1.01	1	13.00	5	0.3186	125
Underground railway	50	757.29	15	9.54	1	12.00	9	5.4800	6,750
Collective urban transport	50	132.00	20	16.72	3	25.00	10	43.7959	30,000
Air transport	50	191.00	30	38.04	15	156.00	3	0.1939	67,500
Railway transport	40	80.00	30	32.09	15	183.00	10	17.1269	180,000
Regular coach services	30	52.00	30	57.32	15	258.00	8	1.1432	108.000
Freight transport									
Courier parcel delivery services	5	3.00	5	1.25	0.1	3.65	8	1.7670	20
Food delivery (catering)	5	3.00	3	0.51	0.1	2.83	7	0.5493	10.5
Grocery delivery	5	3.00	3	0.51	2	16.67	5	0.3114	150
Heavy transport	0.5	2.00	7	3.75	3	24.00	8	3.0408	84

Having compared the results collated in Tables 6.7 and 6.8, one should note the significant impact of the restrictions and constraints related to the mask use and social distancing obligations (the carrying capacity of means of transport limited to a half) on the results of the transport-associated epidemic risk assessment. In all cases, except for the car sharing service whose very nature results in the absence of a direct impact of those restrictions on the risk of infection, the R_{eT} value has been found to increase considerably. This has resulted in reclassification of the risk level for taxi services and grocery deliveries from negligible to low, and placed collective public transport services at the significant risk level. With regard to passenger rail, air and coach transport, the level of epidemic risk has risen to the very high and unacceptable level.

Additionally, also the effect of individual transport process variants categorised under representative groups of transport services, as described in Chapter 4, on the epidemic risk assessment results and the R_{eT} coefficient values has been analysed. The analysis results are provided in Table 6.9. It should be highlighted that only differing values of viral pathogen transmission probability, characteristic to the given process of provision of different transport service variants, have been taken into account in this analysis. When developing service delivery variants under the conditions of various epidemic threats, causing the number of exposed persons or the time of exposure to the pathogen to decline, the R_{eT} risk assessment values may change even more towards the risk level reduction. The relevant cells in the table are analogically marked with greyscales representing the risk levels identified in Table 6.3.

Additionally, mean values of the risk levels and the standard deviation from the mean value of R_{eT} as well as the variants for which the risk level is the lowest and the highest have been established, as provided in Table 6.10.

Having analysed the simulations performed as well as comparisons and assessment scores thus obtained, one will conclude that the mortality factor established by considering the social and global aspects in the assessment of risk attributable to transport was particularly important for the final risk assessment.

If the risk was to be analysed with regard to a single transport service only, without taking into account the external effects that affect the development of the epidemic, the mortality factor could be disregarded. Given the huge impact of mobility, and consequently also of the entire transport sector, on the epidemic development, the author strongly advises against such an approach. However, for cognitive purposes, a comparative analysis of the risk assessed for isolated transport services has been performed, and the result provided as the infection risk of a single person participating in transport.

In this case, formula 6.1 assumes the following form:

$$R_{ei} = P_i \cdot E_i \cdot L_i \tag{6.2}$$

Table 6.9 Summary of the R_{eT} values obtained by assessing the transport-associated epidemic risk for different variants of the service provision process

Epidemic risk in transport R_{eT}	Variant 1		Variant 2		Variant 3		Variant 4		Variant 5		Variant 6	
	Mask	No mask	Mask	No mask	Mask	No mask	Mask	No mask	Mask	No mask	Mask	No mask
Passenger transport												
Car sharing	1.5	4.5	0.75	4.5	0.75	0.75						
Taxi	5	15	5	15								
Underground railway	2,450	5,250	2,450	5,250	2,450	5,250	2,450	5,250				
Collective urban transport	9,450	18,900	9,450	18,900	9,450	18,900	9,450	18,900				
Air transport	11,250	18,750	11,250	18,750	11,250	18,750	11,250	18,750		18,750	11,250	18,750
Railway transport	48,000	72,000	48,000	72,000								
Regular coach service	13,500	20,250	13,500	20,250								
Freight transport												
Courier parcel delivery services	1	1	2	6	2	10						
Food delivery (catering)	0.5	3	0.5	3								
Grocery delivery	5	30	5	30								
Heavy transport	45	63	4.5	4.5								

Table 6.10 Summary of the statistical values of coefficient R_{eT} obtained by assessing the transport-associated epidemic risk for different variants of the service provision process

Epidemic risk in transport R_{eT}	R_{eT} median	STD	R_{eT} min.	R_{eT} max.
Passenger transport				
Car sharing	1.125	1.70	0.75	4.5
Taxi	10	5	5	15
Underground railway	3,850	1,400	2,450	5,250
Collective urban transport	14,175	4,725	9,450	18,900
Air transport	15,000	3,750	11,250	18,750
Railway transport	60,000	12,000	48,000	72,000
Regular coach service	16,875	3,375	13,500	20,250
Freight transport				
Courier parcel delivery services	1.5	3.40	1	10
Food delivery (catering)	1.75	1.25	0.5	3
Grocery delivery	17.5	12.5	5	30
Heavy transport	24.75	25.56	4.5	63

where:

P_i – probability of viral pathogen transmission attributable to the ith transport service (Table 4.19),

E_i – exposure time, i.e. mean time of direct contact between participants of the ith transport process,

L_i – number of potentially infectious persons, i.e. the number of persons involved in a chain of events within a certain unit of time of process implementation (30 min).

The values of coefficient R_{ei} range between 0.005 and 22,500.

As implied by the analysis of this case, it is also possible to assume the number of exposed persons as the number of potentially infectious persons, analogically to formula 6.1.

Having computed the analysed cases, one obtains the viral infection risk assessment for a single provision of a transport service, i.e. R_{ei}. A summary similar to those in Tables 6.7 and 6.8 for the values of R_{eT} is provided in Table 6.11, this one considering the current restrictions and the obligation to wear protective masks and maintain social distance (principle of using 50% capacity of means of transport).

The foregoing clearly implies that an individualised approach to risk assessment, in separation from its global effects, causes the hierarchy of transport services to change. In terms of viral infection, the most dangerous means of transport seem to be passenger air transport followed by rail and coach transport. The viral infection risk considered in the absence of any

Table 6.11 Comparison of infection risks R_{ei} for a single transport service provision, considering cases with and without restrictions

Infection risk in transport	No. of exposed persons	Transmission probability (%)	Exposure time	R_{ei}	No. of exposed persons	Transmission probability (%)	Exposure time	R_{ei}
Passenger transport	With interventions and restrictions				No interventions and restrictions			
Car sharing	0.5	0.5	3	**0.75**	0.5	0.5	3	**0.75**
Taxi	5	3	1	**15**	5	5	1	**25**
Underground railway	50	10	1	**500**	50	15	1	**750**
Collective urban transport	35	15	3	**1,575**	50	20	3	**3,000**
Air transport	50	20	15	**15,000**	50	30	15	**22,500**
Railway transport	20	25	15	**7,500**	40	30	15	**18,000**
Regular coach service	15	25	15	**5,625**	30	30	15	**13,500**
Freight transport								
Courier parcel delivery services	5	1	0.1	**0.5**	5	5	0.1	**2.5**
Food delivery (catering)	5	1	0.1	**0.5**	5	3	0.1	**1.5**
Grocery delivery	5	1	2	**10**	5	3	2	**30**
Heavy transport	0.5	3	3	**4.5**	0.5	7	3	**10.5**

restrictions imposed on air transport reaches even up to the maximum level of 22,500, which is the upper threshold of the rating scale based on the R_{ei} values. The hierarchy also changes in freight transport, where on account of the R_{ei} value the most risky service appears to be grocery delivery.

6.5 CONCLUSIONS

Comprehensive assessment of the epidemic risk attributable to transport is somewhat a novelty, going far beyond the earlier approach that boils down to establishing the viral infection probability for specific means of transport.

The comprehensive method developed by the author for purposes of transport-associated epidemic risk assessment enables a quantitative and fully explicit risk assessment. The analysis of the results previously obtained, based on an expert assessment of the epidemic risk in transport and the information on the spread of the SARS-CoV-2 virus pandemic acquired to date, implies that the assumptions originally made and the analytical method adopted are both correct. The components of the multiplicative R_{eT} coefficient, as proposed by the author, are important determinants of the transport-associated epidemic risk assessment. The partial factor scales established for purposes of the analysis are non-linear in nature, and strongly correlated with the characteristics of the distribution of values across the entire transport sector with regard to representative groups of services. This made it possible to achieve a satisfactory correlation for the sensitivity of the effects of the partial factors on the final epidemic risk factor. The foregoing has been confirmed by multiple variant analyses, synthetically described in this chapter. Correctness of the thresholds proposed for the values of the R_{eT} epidemic risk coefficient, being the very foundation of the risk level classification, can also be confirmed. Using the fully explicit mathematical notation of the author's signature risk assessment method, one should apply the operational algorithms dedicated to the methods intended for determining the partial measures described in Chapters 4 and 5.

The comprehensive multi-criteria method of transport-associated epidemic risk assessment proposed by the author also provides the grounds for epidemic risk management in transport. The originally defined risk levels were considered against the recommended risk management strategies, thus providing a starting point for designing a comprehensive epidemic risk management system for transport.

Additionally, given the assumption that a generic approach should be applied to the risk assessment in light of the national epidemic situation, the method in question can also serve the purposes of studies of the epidemic risk management of the given country.

For illustrative purposes, the author has also proposed the R_{ei} coefficient for the assessment of transport-associated risk with reference to a single person. However, given the importance of the transport sector as a social and economic mobility platform, the author strongly recommends that one should apply the methodology based on the R_{eT} coefficient which determines the level of epidemic risk attributable to transport.

When considering the epidemic risk management limited to the sphere of a chosen transport company, this methodology can be used to select or design an optimal variant of transport service delivery.

Chapter 7

Conclusion

The subject matter of this book entitled *Epidemic Risk Analysis and Assessment in Transport Services: COVID-19 and Other Viruses* is very topical in the first place, but also interesting in cognitive terms and very relevant from a practical perspective. At the same time, being fully aware of the underlying responsibility and practicality of the methodology proposed, this subject can be claimed to represent a great scientific challenge. Even though the overall body of risk management-related concepts has been known and developed for many years all over the world, considering the subject and object of this monograph, namely, the epidemic risk attributable to transport, it most probably constitutes a scientific novelty.

An unquestionable advantage of the methodology proposed by the author is the fully explicit mathematical notation based on quantitative measures, which makes the entire method quantitatively objective in nature. This additionally guarantees universality of the method when used to assess the epidemic risk in transport, provided that analogous input data sets can be compiled. The said universality applies to both the area of application (local, regional, sector-specific or global) and the object of risk analysis, i.e. any kind of epidemic risk. However, this calls for adapting the method to the current state of knowledge regarding the pathogen transmission models and epidemic indicators.

It can also be used as a tool to support forecasting and variant analyses of how the epidemic develops depending on the restrictions imposed on the transport sector.

However, the method primarily provides a foundation for dedicated transport-related risk management systems, which results from numerous reasons, including the comprehensive and complementary nature of the approach it represents.

The first step in the process is identification and assessment of the relevant epidemic threats attributable to transport. It is precisely for this purpose that a method known as Deep Hazard Identification (DHI) has been developed. DHI enables a detailed analysis of threats based on process maps and dedicated quantitative scales intended for assessing the criteria that affect the mechanisms of virus transmission. The DHI index enables quantitative

DOI: 10.1201/9781003204732-7

multi-criteria weighted assessment of the epidemic hazard. Consequently, this makes it possible to determine a matrix of epidemic hazard assessment for transport services. Using this method, one can not only build a collective table of hazard factors for a selected group of transport services, but also identify the predominant sources of hazards and compare selected services against the context of the risk involved in epidemic threats. This may provide grounds for making decisions with regard to the choice of transport services or set a hierarchy of goals in the context of minimising or eliminating hazard factors, which is the first step in risk management. This is a fully original signature approach which enables accurate identification and objective (i.e. quantitative) assessment of the epidemic hazards attributable to transport.

Chapter 4 of this monograph presents a novel approach to estimating the probability of viral pathogen transmission for representative groups of transport services by taking several variants of service delivery processes into account. Some of the main strengths of the methodology proposed by the author include its process approach, making it possible to consider factors other than virus transmission only in transport, and the analysis of all mechanisms of virus transmission via droplet and touch routes. When calculating the total probability of viral pathogen transmission in the given transport service, the author referred to the definition of probability of a sum of independent events. When determining the elementary events comprising activities that may involve potential pathogen transmission, the DHI analysis was used. The aggregate summaries of the values of probability of viral pathogen transmission prepared with regard to the chosen groups of services, for different variants of their implementation, make it possible to directly compare the factors which facilitate decision-making, even in light of the substitutive or complementary nature of the transport process.

Subsequently, a methodology for estimating the effects of epidemic threats attributable to transport was proposed with reference to the SARS-CoV-2 virus pandemic. The author originally assumed that, given the enormous impact of mobility, implemented by means of various transport services, on the development of the epidemic, the analysis of the effects of transport-associated infections would refer to the scale of the entire country, and take daily indicators into account. Nevertheless, the methodology developed by the author as a means to estimate the effects of epidemic threats attributable to transport services is universal in nature. Given its complete openness and mathematic formalisation, this method is suitable for application against any chosen criteria. It can be expanded or limited geographically, from the scale of a single municipality to that of the entire world. It can be narrowed down to a specific company or even a single service provision case. Furthermore, the estimation ranges also depend on the nature of the epidemic threat. Statistical indicators were applied in this method. Owing to their open mathematical format it is possible to determine the value of these indicators each time depending on the area of the method application and the epidemic type while trying to obtain analogical data sets. The author has also proposed an interesting data estimation solution, which proves particularly helpful in the absence of detailed real-life data on the transport sector, based on case studies, process maps and chains of events. The methodology proposed for estimation of the effects of viral infection attributable to transport services can significantly complement the methodology of the epidemic evolution studies and represent an important source of knowledge to be used when identifying process-related (non-stationary) epidemic outbreaks.

Chapter 6 describes a comprehensive method of epidemic risk assessment in transport. The method developed by the author enables quantitative and fully explicit risk assessment. A multiplicative factor of R_{eT} was proposed as a risk measure, where the relevant constituent factors are important determinants of the epidemic risk assessment for transport. The scales established for the constituent factors are non-linear in nature and, when considering representative groups of services, they are heavily correlated with the characteristics of the distribution of values across the entire transport sector. For this reason, the sensitivity of the effect of the constituent measures on the final epidemic risk factor could be successfully correlated. Making the most of the fully explicit mathematical notation of the risk assessment method proposed, one should apply the algorithms dedicated to the methods aimed to enable determination of the constituent factors, as described in Chapters 4 and 5. Consequently, the array of methods proposed by the author should be considered as a fully universal methodology for assessment of the epidemic risk in transport, which can be successfully applied in other countries or on a global scale when compiling analogical data sets.

The comprehensive multi-criteria method intended as a means to assess the epidemic risk attributable to transport also provides grounds for the epidemic risk management in transport. Specific risk levels were defined and subsequently correlated with the recommended risk management strategies, thus establishing a starting point for developing a comprehensive system of transport-associated epidemic risk management. For instance, when developing service delivery variants addressing the relevant epidemic threats, ones that can further reduce the number of persons exposed to the pathogen or the exposure time, one should realise that values of the R_{eT} risk assessment factor may change even more than those resulting from the lower infection probability established for the given variant, with the risk value showing a declining trend. To this end, one should proceed in line with the DHI analysis and use the matrix of hazard assessment, both providing valid starting points under the methodology developed by the author.

The methodology proposed for the assessment of the epidemic risk attributable to transport from a comprehensive perspective is a novelty in a sense that it goes far beyond the current approach which boils down to determining the probability of viral infection in specific means of transport.

Moreover, considering the pre-assumed general approach to risk assessment vis-à-vis the national epidemic situation, the method developed by the author of this monograph appears to be suitable for studying epidemic risk management policies of specific countries.

References

Abdussamie, N., Zaghwan, A., Daboos, M., Elferjani, I., Mehanna, A., Su, W., 2018. Operational risk assessment of offshore transport barges. Ocean Eng. 156, 333–346. https://doi.org/10.1016/j.oceaneng.2018.03.006

Arias Velásquez, R.M., Mejía Lara, J.V., 2020a. Forecast and evaluation of COVID-19 spreading in USA with reduced-space Gaussian process regression. Chaos, Solitons and Fractals 136. https://doi.org/10.1016/j.chaos.2020.109924

Arias Velásquez, R.M., Mejía Lara, J.V., 2020b. Gaussian approach for probability and correlation between the number of COVID-19 cases and the air pollution in Lima. Urban Clim. 33. https://doi.org/10.1016/j.uclim.2020.100664

Beigel, J.H., Tomashek, K.M., Dodd, L.E., Mehta, A.K., Zingman, B.S., Kalil, A.C., Hohmann, E., Chu, H.Y., Luetkemeyer, A., Kline, S., Lopez de Castilla, D., Finberg, R.W., Dierberg, K., Tapson, V., Hsieh, L., Patterson, T.F., Paredes, R., Sweeney, D.A., Short, W.R., Touloumi, G., Lye, D.C., Ohmagari, N., Oh, M., Ruiz-Palacios, G.M., Benfield, T., Fätkenheuer, G., Kortepeter, M.G., Atmar, R.L., Creech, C.B., Lundgren, J., Babiker, A.G., Pett, S., Neaton, J.D., Burgess, T.H., Bonnett, T., Green, M., Makowski, M., Osinusi, A., Nayak, S., Lane, H.C., 2020. Remdesivir for the treatment of Covid-19 — Final report. N. Engl. J. Med. 383, 1813–1826. https://doi.org/10.1056/nejmoa2007764

Bęczkowska, S., Grabarek, I., Choromański, W., 2013. A model of risk assessment concerning the road transportation of hazardous materials – selected issues. Prace naukowe Politechniki Warszawskiej, Transport 96, 77–86 (in Polish).

Bogoch, I.I., Watts, A., Thomas-Bachli, A., Huber, C., Kraemer, M.U.G., Khan, K., 2020. Pneumonia of unknown aetiology in Wuhan, China: Potential for international spread via commercial air travel. J. Travel Med. 27, 1–3. https://doi.org/10.1093/jtm/taaa008

Böhmer, M.M., Buchholz, U., Corman, V.M., Hoch, M., Katz, K., Marosevic, D.V., Böhm, S., Woudenberg, T., Ackermann, N., Konrad, R., Eberle, U., Treis, B., Dangel, A., Bengs, K., Fingerle, V., Berger, A., Hörmansdorfer, S., Ippisch, S., Wicklein, B., Grahl, A., Pörtner, K., Muller, N., Zeitlmann, N., Boender, T.S., Cai, W., Reich, A., Van der Heiden, M., Rexroth, U., Hamouda, O., Schneider, J., Veith, T., Mühlemann, B., Wölfel, R., Antwerpen, M., Walter, M., Protzer, U., Liebl, B., Haas, W., Sing, A., Drosten, C., Zapf, A., 2020. Investigation of a COVID-19 outbreak in Germany resulting from a single travel-associated primary case: a case series. Lancet Infect. Dis. 20, 920–928. https://doi.org/10.1016/S1473-3099(20)30314-5

Boone, S.A., Gerba, C.P., 2007. Significance of fomites in the spread of respiratory and enteric viral disease. Appl. Environ. Microbiol. 73, 1687–1696. https://doi.org/10.1128/AEM.02051-06

Brok, J., 1998. 4P Teoria granicy iloczynu Kaplana-Meiera w analizie przeżycia. Reports Pract. Oncol. Radiother. 3, 42. https://doi.org/10.1016/s1507-1367(98)70216-0

Burdzik, R., Ciesla, M., Sładkowski, A., 2014. Cargo loading and unloading efficiency analysis in multimodal transport. Promet – Traffic – Traffico 26, 323–331. https://doi.org/10.7307/ptt.v26i4.1356

Chen, S., Owolabi, Y., Li, A., Lo, E., Robinson, P., Janies, D., Lee, C., Dulin, M., 2020. Patch dynamics modeling framework from pathogens' perspective: Unified and standardized approach for complicated epidemic systems. PLoS One 15. https://doi.org/10.1371/journal.pone.0238186

Chen, S., Yang, J., Yang, W., Wang, C., Bärnighausen, T., 2020. COVID-19 control in China during mass population movements at New Year. Lancet 395, 764–766. https://doi.org/10.1016/S0140-6736(20)30421-9

Chen, Y.-C., Lu, P.-E., Chang, C.-S., Liu, T.-H., 2020. A time-dependent SIR model for COVID-19 with undetectable infected persons. IEEE Trans. Netw. Sci. Eng. 1–1. https://doi.org/10.1109/tnse.2020.3024723

Colubri, A., Yadav, K., Jha, A., Sabeti, P.C., 2020. Individual-level modeling of COVID-19 epidemic risk. arXiv Preprint.

Dai, H., Zhao, B., 2020. Association of infected probability of COVID-19 with ventilation rates in confined spaces: A Wells-Riley equation based investigation. https://doi.org/10.1101/2020.04.21.20072397

Ferretti, L., Wymant, C., Kendall, M., Zhao, L., Nurtay, A., Abeler-Dörner, L., Parker, M., Bonsall, D., Fraser, C., 2020. Quantifying SARS-CoV-2 transmission suggests epidemic control with digital contact tracing. Science (80-.) 368, 0–8. https://doi.org/10.1126/science.abb6936

Fine, J.P., Gray, R.J., 1999. A proportional hazards model for the subdistribution of a competing risk. J. Am. Stat. Assoc. 94, 496–509. https://doi.org/10.1080/01621459.1999.10474144

Flaxman, S., Mishra, S., Gandy, A., Juliette, H., Unwin, T., Coupland, H., Mellan, T.A., Zhu, H., Berah, T., Eaton, J.W., Guzman, P.N.P., Schmit, N., Callizo, L., Whittaker, C., Winskill, P., Xi, X., Ghani, A., Donnelly, C.A., Riley, S., Okell, L.C., Vollmer, M.A.C., Ferguson, N.M., Bhatt, S., 2020. Estimating the number of infections and the impact of non-pharmaceutical interventions on COVID-19 in European countries: Technical description update. arXiv, 1–7.

Fridstrøm, L., 2020. Who will bell the cat? On the environmental and sustainability risks of electric vehicles: A comment. Transp. Res. Part A Policy Pract. 135, 354–357. https://doi.org/10.1016/j.tra.2020.03.017

Garciá De Abajo, F.J., Hernández, R.J., Kaminer, I., Meyerhans, A., Rosell-Llompart, J., Sanchez-Elsner, T., 2020. Back to normal: An old physics route to reduce SARS-CoV-2 transmission in indoor spaces. ACS Nano 14, 7704–7713. https://doi.org/10.1021/acsnano.0c04596

Ghani, A.C., Donnelly, C.A., Cox, D.R., Griffin, J.T., Fraser, C., Lam, T.H., Ho, L.M., Chan, W.S., Anderson, R.M., Hedley, A.J., Leung, G.M., 2005. Methods for estimating the case fatality ratio for a novel, emerging infectious disease. Am. J. Epidemiol. 162, 479–486. https://doi.org/10.1093/aje/kwi230

Gogolewski, K., Rosińska M., Rabczenko, D., Szczurek, E., Miasojedow, B., Gambin, A., 2020. COVID-19 model on-line. MIMUW (https://covid19. mimuw.edu.pl/analiza_smiertelnosci.html)

Goshua, G., Pine, A.B., Meizlish, M.L., Chang, C.H., Zhang, H., Bahel, P., Baluha, A., Bar, N., Bona, R.D., Burns, A.J., Dela Cruz, C.S., Dumont, A., Halene, S., Hwa, J., Koff, J., Menninger, H., Neparidze, N., Price, C., Siner, J.M., Tormey, C., Rinder, H.M., Chun, H.J., Lee, A.I., 2020. Endotheliopathy in COVID-19-associated coagulopathy: Evidence from a single-centre, cross-sectional study. Lancet Haematol. 7, e575–e582. https://doi.org/10.1016/S2352-3026(20)30216-7

Guerrero, N., Brito, J., Cornejo, P., 2020. COVID-19. Transport of respiratory droplets in a microclimatologic urban scenario 1–5. https://doi.org/10.1101/2020.04.17.20064394

Haight, F.A., 1986. Risk, especially risk of traffic accident. Accid. Anal. Prev. 18, 359–366. https://doi.org/10.1016/0001-4575(86)90009-6

Harvey, A.P., Fuhrmeister, E.R., Cantrell, M.E., Pitol, A.K., Swarthout, J.M., Powers, J.E., Nadimpalli, M.L., Julian, T.R., Pickering, A.J., 2021. Longitudinal monitoring of SARS-CoV-2 RNA on high-touch surfaces in a community setting. Environ. Sci. Technol. Lett. 8(2), 168–175.

Hauer, E., 1982. Traffic conflicts and exposure. Accid. Anal. Prev. 14, 359–364. https://doi.org/10.1016/0001-4575(82)90014-8

He, S., Peng, Y., Sun, K., 2020. SEIR modeling of the COVID-19 and its dynamics. Nonlinear Dyn. 101, 1667–1680. https://doi.org/10.1007/s11071-020-05743-y

He, X., Lau, E.H.Y., Wu, P., Deng, X., Wang, J., Hao, X., Lau, Y.C., Wong, J.Y., Guan, Y., Tan, X., Mo, X., Chen, Y., Liao, B., Chen, W., Hu, F., Zhang, Q., Zhong, M., Wu, Y., Zhao, L., Zhang, F., Cowling, B.J., Li, F., Leung, G.M., 2020. Temporal dynamics in viral shedding and transmissibility of COVID-19. Nat. Med. 26, 672–675. https://doi.org/10.1038/s41591-020-0869-5

Hellewell, J., Abbott, S., Gimma, A., Bosse, N.I., Jarvis, C.I., Russell, T.W., Munday, J.D., Kucharski, A.J., Edmunds, W.J., Sun, F., Flasche, S., Quilty, B.J., Davies, N., Liu, Y., Clifford, S., Klepac, P., Jit, M., Diamond, C., Gibbs, H., van Zandvoort, K., Funk, S., Eggo, R.M., 2020. Feasibility of controlling COVID-19 outbreaks by isolation of cases and contacts. Lancet Glob. Heal. 8, e488–e496. https://doi.org/10.1016/S2214-109X(20)30074-7

Hopfe, C.J., Augenbroe, G.L.M., Hensen, J.L.M., 2013. Multi-criteria decision making under uncertainty in building performance assessment. Build. Environ. 69, 81–90. https://doi.org/10.1016/j.buildenv.2013.07.019

Hu, M., Lin, H., Wang, J., Xu, C., Tatem, A.J., Meng, B., Zhang, X., Liu, Y., Wang, P., Wu, G., Xie, H., Lai, S., 2020. Risk of coronavirus disease 2019 transmission in train passengers: An epidemiological and modeling study. Clin. Infect. Dis. 1–7. https://doi.org/10.1093/cid/ciaa1057

Johnson, N.P.A.S., Mueller, J., 2002. Updating the accounts: Global mortality of the 1918–1920 "Spanish" influenza pandemic. Bull. Hist. Med. 76, 105–115. https://doi.org/10.1353/bhm.2002.0022

Jordan, E.O., 1927. Epidemic influenza. A survey. Epidemic Influ. A Surv.

Kaplan, E.L. & Meier, P., 1958. Nonparametric estimation from incomplete observations. J. Am. Statist. Assoc., 53:282, 457–481, DOI: 10.1080/01621459.1958.10501452

Karako, K., Song, P., Chen, Y., Tang, W., 2020. Analysis of COVID-19 infection spread in Japan based on stochastic transition model. Biosci. Trends 14, 134–138. https://doi.org/10.5582/bst.2020.01482

Klotz, L., Horman, M., Bi, H.H., Bechtel, J., 2008. The impact of process mapping on transparency. Int. J. Product. Perform. Manag. 57, 623–636. https://doi.org/10.1108/17410400810916053

Ko, G., Thompson, K.M., Nardell, E.A., 2004. Estimation of tuberculosis risk on a commercial airliner. Risk Anal. 24, 379–388. https://doi.org/10.1111/j.0272-4332.2004.00439.x

Krystek, R. 2009. Integrated transport safety system. Warszawa, p. 480 (in Polish).

Kucharski, A.J., Russell, T.W., Diamond, C., Liu, Y., Edmunds, J., Funk, S., Eggo, R.M., Sun, F., Jit, M., Munday, J.D., Davies, N., Gimma, A., van Zandvoort, K., Gibbs, H., Hellewell, J., Jarvis, C.I., Clifford, S., Quilty, B.J., Bosse, N.I., Abbott, S., Klepac, P., Flasche, S., 2020. Early dynamics of transmission and control of COVID-19: A mathematical modelling study. Lancet Infect. Dis. 20, 553–558. https://doi.org/10.1016/S1473-3099(20)30144-4

Kumar, A., Mishra, R.K., 2018. Human health risk assessment of major air pollutants at transport corridors of Delhi, India. J. Transp. Heal. 10, 132–143. https://doi.org/10.1016/j.jth.2018.05.013

Lai, S., Bogoch, I., Ruktanonchai, N., Watts, A., Lu, X., Yang, W., Yu, H., Khan, K., Tatem, A., 2020. Assessing spread risk of Wuhan novel coronavirus within and beyond China, January-April 2020: A travel network-based modelling study. medRxiv Prepr. Serv. Heal. Sci. https://doi.org/10.1101/2020.02.04.20020479

Lavezzo, E., Franchin, E., Ciavarella, C., Cuomo-Dannenburg, G., Barzon, L., Del Vecchio, C., Rossi, L., Manganelli, R., Loregian, A., Navarin, N., Abate, D., Sciro, M., Merigliano, S., Decanale, E., Vanuzzo, M.C., Saluzzo, F., Onelia, F., Pacenti, M., Parisi, S., Carretta, G., Donato, D., Flor, L., Cocchio, S., Masi, G., Sperduti, A., Cattarino, L., Salvador, R., Gaythorpe, K., Brazzale, A., Toppo, S., Trevisan, M., Baldo, V., Donnelly, C., Ferguson, N., Dorigatti, I., Crisanti, A., 2020. Suppression of COVID-19 outbreak in the municipality of Vo, Italy. Nature 1–23. https://doi.org/10.1101/2020.04.17.20053157

Lewis, R.C., Rauschenberger, R., Kalmes, R., 2020. Hand-to-mouth and other hand-to-face touching behavior in a quasi-naturalistic study under controlled conditions. J. Toxicol. Environ. Heal. – Part A 84(2), 49–55. https://doi.org/10.1080/15287394.2020.1830457

Librantz, A., Santos, F., Dias, C., Cunha, A., Costa, I., Librantz, A., Santos, F., Dias, C., Cunha, A., Costa, I., Modelling, A.H.P., 2017. AHP modelling and sensitivity analysis for evaluating the criticality of software programs In: Nääs I. et al. (eds) Advances in Production Management Systems. Initiatives for a Sustainable World. APMS 2016. IFIP Advances in Information and Communication Technology, vol 488. Springer, Cham. https://doi.org/10.1007/978-3-319-51133-7_30.

Lu, J., Gu, J., Li, K., Xu, C., Su, W., Lai, Z., ... & Yang, Z. (2020). COVID-19 outbreak associated with air conditioning in restaurant, Guangzhou, China, 2020. *Emerging infectious diseases*, 26(7), 1628.

Mangili, A., Gendreau, M.A., 2005. Transmission of infectious diseases during commercial air travel. Lancet 365, 989–996. https://doi.org/10.1016/S0140-6736(05)71089-8

Mahsin, M.D., Deardon, R., Brown, P., 2020. Geographically dependent individual-level models for infectious diseases transmission. Biostatistics, kxaa009.https://doi.org/10.1093/biostatistics/kxaa009

Melikov, A.K., Ai, Z.T., Markov, D.G., 2020. Intermittent occupancy combined with ventilation: An efficient strategy for the reduction of airborne transmission indoors. Sci. Total Environ. 744. https://doi.org/10.1016/j.scitotenv.2020.140908

Mouchtouri, V.A., Koureas, M., Kyritsi, M., Vontas, A., Kourentis, L., Sapounas, S., Rigakos, G., Petinaki, E., Tsiodras, S., Hadjichristodoulou, C., 2020. Environmental contamination of SARS-CoV-2 on surfaces, air-conditioner and ventilation systems. Int. J. Hyg. Environ. Health 230, 113599. https://doi.org/10.1016/j.ijheh.2020.113599

Mukhra, R., Krishan, K., Kanchan, T., 2020. Possible modes of transmission of novel coronavirus SARS-CoV-2: A review. Acta Biomed. https://doi.org/10.23750/abm.v91i3.10039

Nande, A., Adlam, B., Sheen, J., Levy, M., Hill, A., 2020. Dynamics of COVID-19 under social distancing measures are driven by transmission network structure. medRxiv Prepr. Serv. Heal. Sci. https://doi.org/10.1101/2020.06.04.20121673

Ng, M.-Y., Wan, E.Y.F., Wong, H.Y.F., Leung, S.T., Lee, J.C.Y., Chin, T.W.-Y., Lo, C.S.Y., Lui, M.M.-S., Chan, E.H.T., Fong, A.H.-T., Yung, F.S., Ching, O.H., Chiu, K.W.-H., Chung, T.W.H., Vardhanbhuti, V., Lam, H.Y.S., To, K.K.W., Chiu, J.L.F., Lam, T.P.W., Khong, P.L., Liu, R.W.T., Man Chan, J.W., Ka Lun Alan, W., Lung, K.-C., Hung, I.F.N., Lau, C.S., Kuo, M.D., Ip, M.S.-M., 2020. Development and validation of risk prediction models for COVID-19 positivity in a hospital setting. Int. J. Infect. Dis. https://doi.org/10.1016/j.ijid.2020.09.022

Olsen, S.J., Chang, H.-L., Cheung, T.Y.-Y., Tang, A.F.-Y., Fisk, T.L., Ooi, S.P.-L., Kuo, H.-W., Jiang, D.D.-S., Chen, K.-T., Lando, J., Hsu, K.-H., Chen, T.-J., Dowell, S.F., 2003. Transmission of the severe acute respiratory syndrome on aircraft. N. Engl. J. Med. 349, 2416–2422. https://doi.org/10.1056/nejmoa031349

Ong, S.W.X., Tan, Y.K., Chia, P.Y., Lee, T.H., Ng, O.T., Wong, M.S.Y., Marimuthu, K., 2020. Air, surface environmental, and personal protective equipment contamination by severe acute respiratory syndrome coronavirus 2 (SARS-CoV-2) from a symptomatic patient. JAMA – J. Am. Med. Assoc. 323, 1610–1612. https://doi.org/10.1001/jama.2020.3227

Patients, L., Taylor, D., Lindsay, A.C., Halcox, J.P., 2020. Correspondence Niacin Compared with Ezetimibe. N. Engl. J. Med. 0–3.

Pitol, A.K., Julian, T.R., 2020. Community transmission of SARS-CoV-2 by fomites: Risks and risk reduction strategies. medRxiv 2020.11.20.20220749.

Polishchuk, V., Kelemen, M., Gavurová, B., Varotsos, C., Andoga, R., Gera, M., Christodoulakis, J., Soušek, R., Kozuba, J., Hospodka, J., Blišťan, P., Szabo, S., 2019. A fuzzy model of risk assessment for environmental start-up projects in the air transport sector. Int. J. Environ. Res. Public Health 16. https://doi.org/10.3390/ijerph16193573

Purdy, G., 2010. ISO 31000:2009 – Setting a new standard for risk management: Perspective. Risk Anal. 30, 881–886. https://doi.org/10.1111/j.1539-6924.2010.01442.x

Riddell, S., Goldie, S., Hill, A., Eagles, D., Drew, T.W., 2020. The effect of temperature on persistence of SARS-CoV-2 on common surfaces. Virol. J. 17, 1–7. https://doi.org/10.1186/s12985-020-01418-7

Riley, E.C., Murphy, G., Riley, R.L. 1978. Airborne spread of measles in a suburban elementary school. Am. J. Epidemiol., 107(5), 421–432.

Rule, A.M., 2020. COVID-19 outbreak associated with air conditioning in restaurant, Guangzhou, China, 2020. Emerg. Infect. Dis. 26, 2791. https://doi.org/10.3201/eid2611.202948

Russell, T.W., Hellewell, J., Jarvis, C.I., Zandvoort, K. Van, Abbott, S., Ratnayake, R., Flasche, S., Eggo, R.M., Edmunds, W.J., Kucharski, A.J., 2020. Estimating the infection and case fatality ratio for coronavirus disease (COVID-19) using age-adjusted data from the outbreak on the Diamond Princess cruise ship, February 2020. Eurosurveillance 25, 6–10. https://doi.org/10.2807/1560-7917.ES.2020.25.12.2000256

Ryan, M.O., Haas, C.N., Gurian, P.L., Gerba, C.P., Panzl, B.M., Rose, J.B., 2014. Application of quantitative microbial risk assessment for selection of microbial reduction targets for hard surface disinfectants. Am. J. Infect. Control 42, 1165–1172. https://doi.org/10.1016/j.ajic.2014.07.024

Saaty, T.L., 2005. Theory and applications of the analytic network process: Decision making with benefits, opportunities, costs, and risks. RWS Publications. Pittsburgh USA.

Saaty, T.L., 2008. Decision Making with the Analytic Hierarchy Process. Int. J. Serv. Sci. 1(1), 83–98.

Schultz, M., Fuchte, J., 2020. Evaluation of aircraft boarding scenarios considering reduced transmissions risks. Sustain. 12. https://doi.org/10.3390/su12135329

Shafaghi, A.H., Rokhsar Talabazar, F., Koşar, A., Ghorbani, M., 2020a. On the effect of the respiratory droplet generation condition on COVID-19 transmission. Fluids 5, 113. https://doi.org/10.3390/fluids5030113

Shafaghi, A.H., Talabazar, F.R., Koşar, A., Ghorbani, M., 2020b. On the effect of the respiratory droplet generation condition on COVID-19 transmission. Fluids. https://doi.org/10.3390/fluids5030113

Sheehan, B., Murphy, F., Mullins, M., Ryan, C., 2019. Connected and autonomous vehicles: A cyber-risk classification framework. Transp. Res. Part A Policy Pract. 124, 523–536. https://doi.org/10.1016/j.tra.2018.06.033

Smieszek, T., 2009. A mechanistic model of infection: Why duration and intensity of contacts should be included in models of disease spread. Theor. Biol. Med. Model. 6. https://doi.org/10.1186/1742-4682-6-25

Smieszek, T., Fiebig, L., Scholz, R.W., 2009. Models of epidemics: When contact repetition and clustering should be included. Theor. Biol. Med. Model. 6. https://doi.org/10.1186/1742-4682-6-11

Smieszek, T., Lazzari, G., Salathé, M., 2019. Assessing the dynamics and control of droplet- and aerosol-transmitted influenza using an indoor positioning system. Sci. Rep. 9. https://doi.org/10.1038/s41598-019-38825-y

Sousa, G.J.B., Garces, T.S., Cestari, V.R.F., Florêncio, R.S., Moreira, T.M.M., Pereira, M.L.D., 2020. Mortality and survival of COVID-19. Epidemiol. Infect. 5–10. https://doi.org/10.1017/S0950268820001405

Sun, C., Zhai, Z., 2020. The efficacy of social distance and ventilation effectiveness in preventing COVID-19 transmission. Sustain. Cities Soc. 62, 102390. https://doi.org/10.1016/j.scs.2020.102390

Tang, B., Wang, X., Li, Q., Bragazzi, N.L., Tang, S., Xiao, Y., Wu, J., 2020. Estimation of the transmission risk of the 2019-nCoV and its implication for public health interventions. J. Clin. Med. 9, 462. https://doi.org/10.3390/jcm9020462

Tian, H., Liu, Y., Li, Y., Wu, C.H., Chen, B., Kraemer, M.U.G., Li, B., Cai, J., Xu, B., Yang, Q., Wang, B., Yang, P., Cui, Y., Song, Y., Zheng, P., Wang, Q., Bjornstad, O.N., Yang, R., Grenfell, B.T., Pybus, O.G., Dye, C., 2020. An investigation of transmission control measures during the first 50 days of the COVID-19 epidemic in China. Science (80-.). 368, 638–642. https://doi.org/10.1126/science.abb6105

Verity, R., Okell, L., Dorigatti, I., Winskill, P., Whittaker, C., Imai, N., Cuomo-Dannenburg, G., Thompson, H., Walker, P.G., Fu, H., Dighe, A., Griffin, J., Baguelin, M., Bhatia, S., Boonyasiri, A., Cori, A., Cucunubá, Z., FitzJohn, R., Gaythorpe, K., Green, W., Hamlet, A., Hinsley, W., Laydon, D., Nedjati-Gilani, G., Riley, S., van Elsland, S., Volz, E., Wang, H., Wang, Y., Xi, X., Donnelly, C., Ghani, A., Ferguson, N., 2020. Estimates of the severity of COVID-19 disease. https://doi.org/10.1101/2020.03.09.20033357

Walker, P.G.T., Whittaker, C., Watson, O.J., Baguelin, M., Winskill, P., Hamlet, A., Djafaara, B.A., Cucunubá, Z., Mesa, D.O., Green, W., Thompson, H., Nayagam, S., Ainslie, K.E.C., Bhatia, S., Bhatt, S., Boonyasiri, A., Boyd, O., Brazeau, N.F., Cattarino, L., Cuomo-Dannenburg, G., Dighe, A., Donnelly, C.A., Dorigatti, I., Van Elsland, S.L., FitzJohn, R., Fu, H., Gaythorpe, K.A.M., Geidelberg, L., Grassly, N., Haw, D., Hayes, S., Hinsley, W., Imai, N., Jorgensen, D., Knock, E., Laydon, D., Mishra, S., Nedjati-Gilani, G., Okell, L.C., Unwin, H.J., Verity, R., Vollmer, M., Walters, C.E., Wang, H., Wang, Y., Xi, X., Lalloo, D.G., Ferguson, N.M., Ghani, A.C., 2020. The impact of COVID-19 and strategies for mitigation and suppression in low- And middle-income countries. Science (80-.) 369, 413–422. https://doi.org/10.1126/science.abc0035

Wilde, G.J.S., 1988. Risk homeostasis theory and traffic accidents: Propositions, deductions and discussion of dissension in recent reactions. Ergonomics 31, 441–468.

Wilde, G.J.S., 1994. Target risk: Dealing with the danger of death, disease and damage in everyday decisions. Toronto: PDE Publications.

Wilde, G.J.S., 1998. Risk homeostasis theory: An overview. Inj. Prev. 4, 89–91. https://doi.org/10.1136/ip.4.2.89

World Health Organization, 2020. Modes of transmission of virus causing COVID-19: Implications for IPC precaution recommendations. Geneva World Heal. Organ. 19–21. https://doi.org/10.1056/NEJMc2004973.Cheng

Xie, X., Li, Y., Chwang, A.T.Y., Ho, P.L., Seto, W.H., 2007. How far droplets can move in indoor environments – revisiting the Wells evaporation-falling curve. Indoor Air 17, 211–225. https://doi.org/10.1111/j.1600-0668.2007.00469.x

Zhang, N., Li, Y., 2018. Transmission of influenza a in a student office based on realistic person-to-person contact and surface touch behaviour. Int. J. Environ. Res. Public Health 15. https://doi.org/10.3390/ijerph15081699

Zhang, X., Ji, Z., Yue, Y., Liu, H., Wang, J., 2020. Infection risk assessment of COVID-19 through aerosol transmission: A case study of South China seafood market. Environ. Sci. Technol. https://doi.org/10.1021/acs.est.0c02895

Index

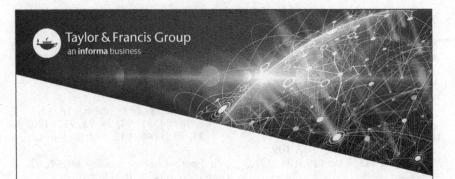